promoting wellness

for Advanced Prostate Cancer Patients, 5th Edition

Your Advanced CSPC to CRPC Empowerment Guide

Mark A. Moyad MD, MPH

SpryPublishing

This edition published by:
Spry Publishing, LLC
326-330 South State Street
Suite 222
Ann Arbor, MI 48104

spry-publishing.com

Printed in the United States of America.

10 9 8 7 6 5 4 3 2 1

ISBN: 978-1-938170-41-6

Dedicated to

This book is dedicated to my dad, Robert H. Moyad, who in my eyes was the finest doctor, father, grandfather, and overall male role model or mentor I was fortunate enough to be around for most of my life. Thank you, Dad, for being you, and I will miss you very much.

It is also dedicated to the other miraculous individuals that changed my life, and those of countless other individuals throughout my 30+ year career—Epstein, Jenkins, Pokempner, and Thompson. Words on a page will never express my appreciation, and the gratitude of the countless individuals out there that benefitted from your kindness.

Another group that deserves recognition are all the oncologists, urologists, nurses, researchers, educators, and all the other healthcare team members from around the world whom I consulted with during the preparation of each edition of this book. I cannot thank you enough for your passion and dedication to your patients, your insatiable appetite to beat cancer, your overall guidance, your objective critiques of each chapter of this book, and your friendship. I am just honored to be a part of this team.

And finally, this book is dedicated to the advocates, advocacy groups, healthcare professionals, patients, partners, and their families who have battled and are still fighting prostate cancer.

Contents

Introduction

WELCOME TO *Promoting Wellness Your Advanced CSPC to CRPC Empowerment Guide, 5th Edition.* Patients and healthcare professionals have made the earlier editions of the book arguably some of the most-utilized informational guides for men, their partners, and overall support team dealing with advanced prostate cancer (AdvPCa), whether it is castrate-sensitive prostate cancer (CSPC), or castrate-resistant prostate cancer (CRPC). In past editions, the term hormone-refractory prostate cancer (HRPC) was used throughout the book, but the term CRPC has become more universally accepted in the medical literature, as well as when searching for the latest information online. Therefore, we decided to exclusively use the term CRPC in this edition (please see "Some Things You Should Know"). With that change, this book could not only be helpful for men and their partners, family members, and medical teams dealing with the different forms of CRPC, including non-metastatic CRPC ("nmCRPC") and metastatic CRPC ("mCRPC"), but also for those dealing with some aspect of "HSPC" (hormone sensitive prostate cancer), which is also known as "CSPC" (castration sensitive prostate cancer). Past and ongoing evidence continues to demonstrate the outstanding potential efficacy and latitude of most CRPC treatments, which appear to work even better when they are introduced earlier in the CRPC process—and now they are even working in some men with HSPC/CSPC!

Along these same lines are the FDA-approved therapies, which continue to grow at a remarkable rate with each new edition. This is incredibly inspiring and should fuel even more optimism in the battle against both CSPC and CRPC! The ongoing amount of positive research recently in this area has been brilliant, and it is coming from all directions now. This includes better medications, better targeted therapies, and better genetic, molecular, or biomarker testing resulting in personalized medicines such as immunotherapy or PARP inhibitors. We are also seeing improved imaging or picture tests, and better prevention and treatment of side effects. There are also more medications working to treat other cancers, which are now being tested and used to treat prostate cancer, as well as more phase 3 clinical trials, more interventions becoming available for compassionate use or expanded access programs (EAPs), and simply more of our wonderful world exceptionally focused on fighting this disease. We have reached a moment in time where we not only have the minds and dedication to solve this puzzle, but also the technology—and that is critical. Will the funding and awareness continue to be there? Yes, I believe this will be the case! Again, reasons for hope and optimism abound.

Interestingly, research has also demonstrated an even better understanding of how lifestyle changes or patient empowerment through knowledge and action can result in a profound difference. In fact, throughout this and other promoting wellness (PW) books we will constantly highlight what I like to call "*PW Lifestyle Empowerment Moments*," to draw ample attention, at last, toward those often unsung educational tips or personalized changes patients can follow to improve their situation. Now, it is time to take it to another level of awareness. Thank you as always for putting your trust in our team and our series of books, which focuses on promoting wellness throughout your journey.

All my best always,

Mark A. Moyad, MD, MPH

P.S. I'd also like to thank our publisher, Jim Edwards, our editor, Robin Porter, and our designer, Anna Herscher for their dedication to these books. It takes a team of talented people to create these valuable resources.

Some Things You Should Know

Before we dive into prognosis indicators and treatment options, it's important to clarify the following topics that can be understandably confusing for many people:

Castrate-Sensitive Prostate Cancer (CSPC) and Castrate-Resistant Prostate Cancer (CRPC)

For advanced prostate cancer still hormone sensitive we will use the term CSPC (castrate-sensitive prostate cancer) or HSPC (hormone-sensitive prostate cancer). When it comes to prostate cancer, CRPC is the most utilized name in the medical literature, and in general, for searches on the Internet, whereas AIPC and HRPC are often less recognized and used today.

Castrate-Resistant Prostate Cancer (CRPC) means the cancer continued to grow and progress even though a man has castrate levels of testosterone (less than 50 ng/dL or 1.7 nmol/L). However, some experts believe the desired level should be less than 20 ng/dL (0.7 nmol/L). Over the years, several names have and continue to be given to imply a situation where PSA rises on traditional androgen deprivation therapy (ADT), such as Androgen-Independent Prostate Cancer (AIPC) and Hormone-Refractory Prostate Cancer (HRPC). However, all these names represented somewhat similar prostate cancer situations (CRPC). For simplicity, we will use CRPC throughout the book because this has become the most-commonly used term, or recognizable name, to access the most up-to-date information online and in medical journals.

Androgen Deprivation Treatment (ADT)

ADT usually continues even after being diagnosed with CRPC. Many men need to continue androgen deprivation treatment (ADT) despite the perception it may no longer be working because it can still help some men with CRPC. Most prostate cancers have an androgen receptor (AR), which is a place where testosterone is accepted or recognized by the tumor(s) so it can grow.

One primary way to stop the tumor is by removing the testosterone that can fit into all those ARs. While this works for many, for others it only works for a limited amount of time. Some men respond for many years to ADT and others respond for a shorter time. Regardless, some preliminary studies suggest that, even if the PSA is rising on ADT, there are still some cancer cells that may respond to testosterone produced by the body. ADT can help eliminate those cancer cells on a regular basis. Research also suggests that there may be a slight reduction in symptoms and a greater survival benefit if a man stays on ADT. Also, it is very important to know that most clinical trials require men to stay on ADT to enroll, so remaining on ADT (ironically also well-known by the term "hormone therapy") keeps options open for your treatment.

Stages 3 and 4 can be really confusing and often misleading non-specific terms.

Stage 3, and especially 4, have been used in some cases to describe a less than optimistic situation, but this is not the case for many men dealing with prostate cancer today.

In fact, these terms are often no longer officially used anymore in many medical circles because they fail to provide more specific or individualized tumor information, including the potential to respond to numerous available treatments. Therefore, these generalized staging terms can underestimate the potential optimism before or during cancer treatment.

The truth is, no one knows your exact prognosis with 100% certainty, because each case is not only different, but every day research takes another step forward, which could suddenly change your prognosis. In fact, this is the most optimistic research period for CSPC/CRPC in history. Multiple treatments have become available for CSPC and CRPC since we started writing this book, with many more options on the verge of becoming available. For example (see the table of contents), there are androgen synthesis inhibitors (abiraterone/Zytiga/Yonsa), second generation anti-androgen pills (apalutamide/Erleada, darolutamide/

Nubeqa, enzalutamide/Xtandi), multiple chemotherapeutic options (docetaxel/Taxotere, cabazitaxel/Jevtana), immune therapies (sipuleucel-T/Provenge, pembrolizumab/Keytruda, etc.), PARP inhibitors (olaparib/Lynparza, rucaparib/Rubraca), radiopharmaceuticals (radium-223/Xofigo), radio-ligand products (lutetium-177), and countless clinical trials available today. Additionally, and probably less appreciated, are some of the recent dramatic advances in prostate cancer imaging, or the ability to now find and more precisely locate prostate cancer wherever it exists throughout the body. Improvements in MRI scans, and in the various types of molecules (choline, fluciclovine, PSMA, etc.) being used in PET/CT scans, for example, should continue to improve the prognosis for many men because they help radiation, or even other drugs, connect with their targets (cancer) with better accuracy than researchers could have ever imagined just a few years ago.

In reality, most men at this stage of the disease can still respond very well to a wide range of options currently available, including many of the medications mentioned earlier. In short, there is no official or specific term in prostate cancer known as a stage 3 or 4 prognosis; and even if there was such a term, the large number of potential AdvPCa treatments available today implies there is tremendous hope and opportunity—not a hopeless situation or a lack of options. The medical team you entrust with your care should be able to provide you with some regular informative or updated guidance on your prognosis, as well as future options.

Advocacy and Support Organizations

The impact of support and advocacy groups on men and their families can be life changing. These groups are some of the most up-to-date resources patients can use for awareness, education, research, clinical trials, drug access, insurance issues, and political advocacy for prostate cancer research.

American Cancer Society
cancer.org

American Society of Clinical Oncology
asco.org

American Urological Association
auanet.org

CancerCare
cancercare.org

Clinical Trials Recruiting, Ongoing & Completed
clinicaltrials.gov

Foundation for Cancer Research and Education
thefcre.org

HRPCa.org
hrpca.org

MaleCare
malecare.org

Man to Man, local groups of the American Cancer Society
cancer.org/treatment/support-programs-and-services.html

National Alliance of State Prostate Cancer Coalitions
naspcc.org

National Comprehensive Cancer Network
nccn.org

Prostate Advocates Aiding Choices in Treatments
paact.help

Prostate Cancer Foundation
pcf.org

Prostate Cancer Info Link
prostatecancerinfolink.net

Prostate Cancer Research and Education Foundation
pcref.org

Prostate Cancer Research Institute (PCRI)
pcri.org

Prostate Conditions Education Council
prostateconditions.org

Prostate Health Education Network, Inc. (PHEN)
prostatehealthed.org

The Prostate Net
prostate.net

Us TOO International Prostate Cancer Education and Support Network
ustoo.org

Zero—The Project to End Prostate Cancer
zerocancer.org

If you live outside of the U.S.—for example in Australia, Canada, or Europe—there are additional outstanding sources of information such as the Prostate Cancer Foundation of Australia, Prostate Cancer Canada, and many others. Please ask your healthcare team about the latest and greatest educational online and other resources for patients.

CHAPTER 1

Understanding & Discussing Prognosis Indicators

35+ Promoting Wellness Tips or Potential Prognosis Indicators from A to Z that You Could Discuss with Your Healthcare Team Before, During or After any Treatment

1. Age

2. Albumin blood test

3. Alkaline phosphatase (ALP) blood test

4. Asymptomatic or symptomatic cancer

5. Bone metastasis and/or number or volume of bone metastasis & oligometastatic prostate cancer (OMPC)

6. Bone-protecting agents (BPAs) & bone healthy behaviors

7. Circulating tumor cell (CTC) blood tests

8. Comorbidities and your medical history/other tests

9. Diet, exercise, sleep quality & quantity, stress reduction, and other lifestyle changes & even OTC medicine interests

10. Germline (your inherited cellular-genetic information since birth) and/or somatic (your cancer) biomarker testing—personalized or precision medicine

11. Gleason total score, Gleason grade group, or primary Gleason score from a pathology report

12. Health disparities, race, ethnicity, & your medical team

13. Hemoglobin/hematocrit/white blood cell/platelet counts-CBC (Complete Blood Count) test & the N:L ratio (bone marrow quality & quantity)

14. Hormone reduction treatment choice (ADT, LHRH, newer daily antagonist pills, or surgical testicular removal)

15. Imaging test results over time— pictures of the inside of the body (bone scan, MRI, PET/CT, etc.) & what and when you eat and exercise (lifestyle) could impact your results

16. Lactate/Lactic Acid Dehydrogenase (LDH) blood test

17. Mental health (stress, anxiety, depression, & associated conditions or issues)

18. Pain	29. Total testosterone (TT) levels before ADT
19. Partner/life partner/support network (it's a couple's disease)	30. Visceral (organs) and/or other soft-tissue disease spread (lymph nodes, organs, organ systems)
20. Performance status (ECOG, etc.)	
21. Preventive vaccines (vaccine preventable Illnesses) for adults including COVID-19	31. Volume (amount) of cancer & quantity/number of sites with cancer—Oligometastatic prostate cancer (OMPC) revisited
22. Previous responses to treatment(s) and/or how well you're able to tolerate treatment(s)	32. Weight loss (excessive/ extreme) or the inability to gain weight when needed
23. Primary tumor site status & treatment, debulking, or "local control" of an advanced cancer	33. You and your medical team Part A. Bi-directional or symbiotic relationship— as important as it gets.
24. PSA & PSA kinetics (PSADT=PSA Doubling Time, PSAV=PSA Velocity, stable PSA, % PSA reductions, etc.)	34. You and your medical team Part B. Even more personalized unique opportunities, access, and assistance with your situation (clinical trials, EAPS, compassion use, appeal letters, insurance issues, etc.)
25. Sarcopenia severity (quality, quantity, & function)	
26. Spiritual health	35. Z = Miscellaneous. Finding health where you and your team did not know it existed.
27. Stage of cancer ("how far it has spread in the body")	
28. Time from initial treatment to AdvPCa, or time on ADT before progressing (converting) to CRPC	36. Bonus. Other Tips or Prognosis Indicators discussed with your medical team & overall support network include:

Promoting Wellness Prognosis Indicators and Educational Tips

The best medical care always begins with good communication. The A-to-Z list of topics above is meant to help you have meaningful and thorough discussions with your healthcare team. Those conversations are easier when you have a list of tests, treatments, assistance and more to reference. Each of the topics on this list are prognosis indicators or factors in determining how someone with advanced prostate cancer (AdvPCa) could do.

Some men have very aggressive AdvPCa, while others have moderately aggressive AdvPCa, and even others, arguably, have more of a mildly aggressive type. Prostate cancer is called a "heterogenous disease" for a good reason. A heterogeneous disease refers to those conditions that have several causes and manifestations, which is why some patients respond well to certain treatments and not so well to others. However, the more treatment opportunities available, then the higher the probability of a good result. Please also bear in mind that no single factor is a clear indicator of success or failure. For example, even when PSA does not respond, or does not respond dramatically, which often occurs with some of the immune therapies or radiopharmaceutical drugs, it can still change a prognosis for the better. Just because one or more of the factors in the next section may be associated with a worse prognosis does not necessarily indicate it will impact your quality and quantity of life. It may mean that discussions with your healthcare team will involve different options appropriate for your individual situation. In other words, knowing that your cancer may be more aggressive can give you a better indication of how aggressively you and your team want to have your cancer treated. Similarly, knowing your cancer may be less aggressive may suggest that a less aggressive approach is needed right now. Please do not be intimidated or overwhelmed by all these potential prognostic factors because they are really educational moments, or opportunities in disguise, to help you and your medical team achieve the highest possible level of communication and success. We will explain each of them.

1. Age

By itself, age has very little impact on whether you would qualify for, or respond to, an AdvPCa treatment. Overall, older men tend to respond just as well as younger men to AdvPCa treatment. In fact, drugs receiving approval for prostate cancer from clinical trials, both in the past and currently, include patients in their 30's and 40's, along with some in their 80's and upper 90's (and every possible age in between), receiving diverse types of treatment. Yet, some men are dealing with more health issues at certain ages (e.g., diabetes, heart disease, other cancers) and this could impact their ability to handle some treatments, which could impact quality and quantity of life.

2. Albumin blood test

Albumin is an important protein. It is the most abundant protein in the blood that is measured by a blood test. Albumin serves as a carrier for all sorts of vital substances in the human body. A normal albumin level is a good indicator that the body is doing well when receiving treatment, while an abnormally low albumin level could be a sign that the patient is not responding as well.

> ### PW Lifestyle Empowerment Moment
>
> There are clinical studies going on right now to see if cancer patients can slightly maintain or increase albumin levels in their blood and help maintain or improve their muscle quality, quantity, and function by increasing or normalizing healthy dietary protein intakes. These studies are interesting, but just starting to get attention. Talk to your medical team, including a dietician, about the latest research. Albumin is not just a marker of nutritional status, but also something that can be reduced by the inflammatory effects of cancer (also known as a "negative acute phase reactant"). Interestingly, many inflammatory markers increase along with body inflammation (known as a "positive acute phase reactant") like C-reactive protein (CRP), which is also a potential

prognostic indicator being studied in prostate cancer. But the albumin laboratory test value tends to decrease with inflammation. Regardless, all of this is a reminder of the importance of discussing lifestyle changes with your healthcare team, even if it has nothing to do with albumin, but rather your overall health and wellness.

3. Alkaline Phosphatase (ALP) blood test

Alkaline Phosphatase is an important enzyme in the body. The ALP blood test measures the amount of this enzyme in the blood, which can help predict the aggressiveness of your AdvPCa, as well as what the cancer is doing to your body. An abnormally high level of this enzyme tends to suggest that the cancer is more aggressive and may not be responding well to the current treatment. ALP (sometimes also abbreviated as just "AP") is mostly made in the liver and bone, but some is also produced in the intestines and kidneys. The level of different forms of ALP in the blood may be measured and used to determine whether an abnormally high level is coming from the liver or bones. This is known as an ALP isoenzymes test. When bone is breaking down at higher-than-normal levels then this test also tends to increase to abnormally higher levels.

PW Lifestyle Empowerment Moment

ALP often decreases when someone is placed on a bone-protective agent (BPA), and it can be reduced with many of the effective AdvPCa direct anti-cancer treatments. Still, it's important to normalize your dietary intake of calcium and vitamin D, and when insufficient, potentially supplement with calcium and vitamin D to make up for the daily difference. Dietary intake of calcium and vitamin D, as well as supplements, were part of the BPA phase 3 clinical trials that led to the FDA approval of drugs such as Xgeva and Zometa. There continues to be debate over the exact need for calcium and vitamin D, but since normalizing daily dietary intake was part of the protocol for these drugs to optimize their effects in preventing bone loss, we can assume calcium and vitamin D play a key role. Normalizing dietary intake of calcium and vitamin D also appeared to have the potential to prevent a rare side effect of these drugs called "hypocalcemia." This is part of the reason calcium and vitamin D are discussed in the actual prescribing information for healthcare professionals when using Xgeva (also known as "denosumab")—the most recent bone drug to be FDA approved for AdvPCa. Not only was vitamin D deficiency associated with hypocalcemia with these bone drugs, a higher ALP level before treatment with a bone drug may also suggest an even higher risk of hypocalcemia. More interesting information on calcium and vitamin D can be found in the next chapter.

4. Asymptomatic or symptomatic

There are two distinctly different clinical situations within AdvPCa; namely, individuals who are asymptomatic (experiencing no symptoms at all) and symptomatic (experiencing some symptoms). Thanks to the PSA test and better imaging tests, the majority of men currently diagnosed with AdvPCa are asymptomatic. This is because the disease is being detected earlier and earlier, opening up more treatment options for AdvPCa patients.
In general, men with asymptomatic AdvPCa have a better prognosis. However, as more drug treatment options for men with symptomatic AdvPCa are becoming available, this may be changing. Many men with symptomatic AdvPCa can become asymptomatic, or at least less symptomatic, if they respond well to these AdvPCa therapies. For example, chemotherapy for CRPC can improve quality-of-life in some AdvPCa patients by reducing symptoms caused by the cancer itself, despite the perception by some people that chemotherapy is associated with worsening quality-of-life. In prostate cancer, many medications, including chemotherapy have the ability to not only improve quantity of life, but also quality by fighting the cancer and delaying its progress, which may prevent or lessen some symptoms.

5. Bone metastasis and/or number, or volume of bone metastasis and oligometastatic prostate cancer (OMPC)

This is somewhat similar to prognostic indicator or educational tip number 31, but also slightly different, because it refers more to cancer spreading to the bones versus other sites. In general, men with AdvPCa who have bone metastasis have a cancer that has usually progressed further than that of someone with no bone metastasis. Individuals with a greater number and/or the size or amount (volume) of bone metastatic spots could have a cancer with a more concerning prognosis. The spine, pelvis, and/or ribs are some of the common sites of metastatic bone spread from prostate cancer. Some research suggests when cancer spreads to less common bone sites, such as the skull or just further away from the spine and pelvic area, then such spread could also be associated with a more advanced or aggressive cancer. The measured amount of space the cancer occupies at one or several bone locations, or in total, is often referred to as the "volume of cancer," which can then be generally referred to as a low- or high-volume cancer. High-volume cancers are more concerning because they occupy more space.

Amazingly, there is a newer and interesting potential prognosis indicator known as "oligometastatic prostate cancer" (OMPC) in some patients. This is a situation where someone has fewer or more localized metastatic spots, versus a larger number and/or more widespread metastatic spots. It appears some men diagnosed with OMPC may have less aggressive advanced tumor(s), or at least respond more favorably to radiation or other treatments when targeted directly at those specific sites. OMPC is an ongoing area of research with multiple different definitions or opinions regarding the number of spots needed to be classified as OMPC (5 or fewer). As this indicator continues to evolve, please also refer to prognostic indicator number 31 later in this chapter. It is similar to the concept introduced earlier of less tumor numbers, or lower tumor volume, which could essentially indicate a better potential prognosis. You should also discuss OMPC with your medical team, which is a far better source of information on your specific prognosis compared to this book.

6. Bone-protecting agents (BPAs) and bone healthy behaviors

The average age of men with prostate cancer puts them at risk for bone loss simply due to aging. Additionally, men with AdvPCa have been or are using ADT, which by itself greatly increases the risk of bone loss and osteoporosis. Lastly, men with AdvPCa are at risk of bone metastasis, which can further increase the risk of several bone problems, including fractures. Therefore, you can see why bone health needs to be a major priority. Bone-protective agents (BPAs) reduce the risk of bone fractures and overall skeletal-related events (SRE), or the problems associated with compromised bone health in many AdvPCa patients whether their risk is from age, ADT, or bone metastasis. Thus, not receiving a BPA in some patients could not only compromise their quality of life, if an SRE occurs, but theoretically impact their prognosis since it could delay effective AdvPCa treatments against the cancer.

PW Lifestyle Empowerment Moment

There are also multiple other bone healthy behaviors, which should be discussed with your healthcare team. For example, inquiring about a simple bone mineral density (BMD) test (for example a DEXA test), normalizing your daily intake of calcium and vitamin D from diet ideally and/or supplements if needed, inquiring about whether weight resistance exercise is an option for you, and other tips can be found in the BPA (Xgeva and Zometa) chapter of this book. The take home message is clear, but it bears repeating—talking to your healthcare team about protecting your bones via medications and lifestyle changes should be a priority.

7. Circulating tumor cells (CTCs) tests

The practice of monitoring circulating tumor cells (CTCs) in the "blood to assess the potential or ongoing effectiveness of a treatment, or provide some indication of prognosis, is starting to get more attention. CTCs are cells that come free or are shed from different tumors and can be found in the blood. These CTCs can be counted in some blood tests, such as "cell search" (see **cellsearchctc.com**). When a drug causes a reduction in CTCs during treatment, or when there are fewer CTCs before the treatment, there could be an improvement in prognosis. This makes sense because a reduction in the number or quantity of tumor cells probably means that some cancer cells have been destroyed.

There are other tests and companies that use CTCs for additional information. For example, there is a fairly new test called "AR-V7" (see **epicsciences.com/ar-v7-test**, **oncotypeiq.com**) that also uses a small amount of blood to determine whether or not you are potentially resistant to androgen receptor (AR) targeted therapies (Erleada, Nubeqa, Xtandi, Zytiga, etc.). Resistance to these treatments suggests a more serious form of prostate cancer. Regardless, whether any of these CTC tests could apply to your situation should be decided by you and your medical team and not this book. Also, see prognostic factor number 10 because personalized genetic, molecular, or simply "biomarker testing" is becoming more common, and could give you more options for CRPC treatment.

8. Comorbidities and your medical history/other tests

It makes sense that your general health and any other diagnosed diseases ("comorbidities") can have an impact on your prognosis. Not surprisingly, individuals with other disease(s) besides prostate cancer could have a more difficult time tolerating some cancer treatments. In addition, these other diseases could shorten a patient's lifespan. Individuals who are healthier in general and who have few to no comorbidities tend to tolerate treatment better and/or simply just live longer. For example, obesity does not seem to dramatically impact AdvPCa prognosis, but it does increase the risk of comorbidities causing health and longevity problems, such as cardiovascular disease or type 2 diabetes, and it also could simply increase the risk of multiple complications from some AdvPCa treatment (fatigue, insulin resistance, nerve damage or neuropathy, etc.). Keeping other diseases and numbers (blood cholesterol, pressure, sugar, etc.) under control as much as possible also protects you from problems arising from other conditions, which could impact your ability to receive timely treatment. Aside from tests related to your cancer, it's important to have other blood tests related to specific organ or body health, such as liver and kidney function tests, because these areas of the body need to be prepared to handle cancer treatment. Thus, whether it is medication compliance to reduce the damaging effects of high blood pressure, and/or putting in more effort at maintaining or improving overall health through lifestyle changes, such as exercise and diet, it makes sense to improve overall quality and quantity of life, which is why we decided to further emphasize it again in the next paragraph and throughout this book.

9. Diet, exercise, sleep quality and quantity, stress reduction, and other lifestyle changes, as well as over-the-counter (OTC) medicine interests

Whether or not any diet or supplements could improve your AdvPCa prognosis specifically has not been proven, but a man who exercises regularly, eats a moderately heart-healthy diet, sleeps with good quality and/or quantity, reduces his stress, and maintains or attempts to maintain a healthy weight/ waist may dramatically improve his quality of life and reduce his risk of other diseases that can reduce his life expectancy. A recent study of men diagnosed with AdvPCa found that a large number of men actually die yearly from other causes, such as cardiovascular disease (CVD), which is the leading cause of death in the U.S. and in most parts of the world. In addition, many prostate cancer treatments have the potential ability to raise cardiovascular risk even further in men high-risk for a cardiovascular event. In other words, not following heart healthy lifestyle changes could cause another problem to surface (e.g., heart attack or stroke) that could further delay your prostate cancer treatment. It should also be emphasized that some OTC products have the potential to reduce quality of life further. For example, some supplements do not combine well with certain types of chemotherapy (see CIPN). Other dietary supplements, such as biotin (vitamin B7) in high dosages, could temporarily interfere with the results of some of your blood tests, including some PSA tests, by artificially increasing or decreasing the results. In the diet and supplement section of the book, you will find heart healthy tips that may fight prostate cancer and improve quality of life. You will also find a list of dietary supplements to consider avoiding or taking based on the latest human or clinical research.

PW Lifestyle Empowerment Moment

Smoking or tobacco use increases the risk of countless diseases, but less known is the ability of smoking to increase the recurrence of many cancers, including prostate cancer, during or after treatment. Smoking also increases the risk of cancer progression, or put more candidly, it encourages some cancers to act more aggressively. It also appears that excessive alcohol intake can do the same thing when it comes to some prostate cancers. If alcohol or tobacco use is an issue for you then please talk to your medical team because there are more ways to help quit than ever before. Interestingly, all these detrimental lifestyle habits are associated with a reduction in sleep quality and quantity, and an increase in acute or chronic stress. However, almost all heart healthy behaviors, such as exercise, eating healthy, not smoking, and moderate-to-no consumption of alcohol could reduce stress (more on this later), as well as improve sleep quality and quantity. Heart Healthy = Sleep Healthy!

10. "Germline" (your inherited cellular-genetic information since birth), and/or "somatic" (from your cancer) biomarker testing—personalized or precision medicine

Genetic or molecular testing for specific mutations in your inherited non-cancerous ("germline") and cancer cells ("somatic") are now being done in men with AdvPCa. In fact, several FDA approved drugs (olaparib, rucaparib, etc.) to treat some prostate and other cancers are an option if a person qualifies based on the results of these tests. Ask your healthcare team if you should be tested for "biomarkers" in your normal/non-cancerous cells, which is also known as "germline testing," and/or in cancer cells from your tumor, which is also known as "somatic testing." Germline testing can be done from a blood sample, inside of mouth/cheek ("buccal swab") or saliva in some cases, and somatic testing can be done from one of your tumor sites (biopsy or surgical tissue), or from portions of cancer cells in your blood (circulating tumor DNA or "ctDNA"). This is also known as a "liquid biopsy." For example, if there is a suggestion of a strong family history of prostate cancer then a genetic mutation known as "BRCA-1" or "BRCA-2" could be responsible for your increased risk of aggressive prostate cancer, and other genetic mutations are being investigated or could be added to this list in time. If you are positive for a mutation associated with more aggressive prostate cancer it is not only potentially informative in your treatment and prognosis, but also for potentially letting your children and other family members (for example brothers and sisters) know if they are also at risk for certain cancers. Regardless, most men with AdvPCa today are also being tested for somatic mutations or molecular changes in their tumor, which can actually change and increase as a cancer evolves with some treatments (also called "acquired" mutations over time), so some men may be tested multiple times before or after different treatments are completed. Again, this is a discussion for you and your medical team because this information is so new. It is becoming more the rule to test men with AdvPCa (or earlier) rather than the exception. The results of these tests could determine whether you qualify for another set of treatments from what is known as PARP inhibitors (olaparib, rucaparib, etc.) to some novel immune therapies and more. There are numerous potential molecular changes, which are potentially "actionable," and could qualify you for a clinical trial or a drug not entertained before in your treatment plan, which is why these tests have become so important. Additional information on this topic is found in the immune and PARP chapters of this book.

Another name for this type of testing matched with specific drug therapies is "personalized or precision medicine biomarker testing." Many laboratories today are not only able to detect actual ctDNA from a liquid biopsy, but also the amount of ctDNA found in your sample ("abundance" or quantity), which could also provide some hint of prognosis in the near future. For example, a higher abundance of ctDNA detected could be associated with a more difficult response to some treatments, and a more challenging prognosis, but at the same time it may better identify a person that could respond to a precision treatment. Again, this is an area of medicine rapidly moving to help patients get more personalized treatment options.

11. Gleason Total Score, Gleason Grade Group, and Primary Gleason Score ("How aggressive was my cancer at diagnosis and how aggressive is it now?")

A higher total Gleason score (scores of 8 to 10, for example) or grade group (4 or 5, for example) when first diagnosed or at a later time indicates a potentially more aggressive cancer. The prognosis or a long-term response to a drug could be more difficult for someone with this type of tumor, as compared with someone who has a moderate or low Gleason score (below 8, for example). Some Gleason scores were established a long time ago for men with a more localized form of this disease, but still knowing these number(s) could be helpful in making treatment decisions. Some researchers believe the first number in your Gleason score, called the primary Gleason score, is as important as the total Gleason score. For example, a primary Gleason score of 4 or 5 suggests a difficult prognosis, as compared to a primary score of 3. A man with a total Gleason score of 5+3=8 may have a worse prognosis, as compared to someone with a score of 4+4=8 in one or several tumor sites.

12. Health Disparities/Race/Ethnicity and Your Medical Team

There are ongoing research debates over the potential specific reasons why some races or minorities, such as African Americans (AA), appear to have more aggressive prostate cancer or lower odds of surviving this disease compared to other groups. Race and ethnicity have an impact on prognosis for many potential researched reasons (e.g., socioeconomics, tumor biology, access to health care services). What is generally not debated is that definitive health disparities truly exist for many individuals today, and it is one the greatest contributors to a potentially worse outcome when diagnosed with many diseases, including prostate cancer. Interestingly, recent comprehensive studies in prostate cancer have suggested, and demonstrated in some cases, that when access to treatment was equal then patients often experienced equal survival advantages. In other words, the lack of access to quality healthcare and delays in adequate treatment are a major obstacle in improving prognosis for many minority groups. If you are in a situation where access to good healthcare is a potential issue then talking to local and national advocacy groups (see this section of the book), your current medical team, including a social worker that could help you access other options, is critical. There are people and groups out there ready to help, and the overlooked or ignored health disparities that are still impacting prognosis needs to change now!

> ### PW Lifestyle Empowerment Moment
>
> Access to more opportunities for physical activity or even access to grocery stores with more healthy food choices are some of the numerous examples of health disparity issues that do not get enough attention. For example, one of the traditional arguments for discouraging healthier food stores or choices was and still is, in some circles, the perceived potential lack of profitability by companies in these locations. This has not been the reality after companies have opened their stores in specific urban and other settings, and in fact profit has profoundly surpassed expectations in numerous areas. Please talk to your extended medical team (social worker, dietician, etc.)

about access suggestions or opportunities in your specific area including the following: healthier food options such as stores, farmer's markets, healthy food distributions centers; free educational classes or lectures offered by the local health center; and a variety of local and national non-profits involved in promoting mental and physical wellness.

13. Hemoglobin/Hematocrit/White Blood Cells/Platelets— Complete Blood Count (CBC) and the N:L ratio (bone marrow quality and quantity)

A hemoglobin count is a measure of the oxygen carrying protein in your red blood cells. If hemoglobin is very low (a condition called "anemia"), a person may feel extremely tired, and it will be more difficult for him to receive treatment. It is not unusual to be slightly anemic due to testosterone-lowering treatment (ADT), but an abnormally low hemoglobin level that causes a variety of symptoms (e.g., fatigue, breathing problems, etc.) may need to be treated. It can make the prognosis slightly worse by causing a delay in cancer treatments. This same story holds true for several other cells produced by your bone marrow and other areas of the body, or those measured from a Complete Blood Count (CBC) test. White blood cells (WBC) come in several different types including the ones that help to primarily fight infections (neutrophils) or those that help with enhancing immune protection (lymphocytes-B & T, etc.). In fact, some medical teams have been looking at the ideal Neutrophil-to-Lymphocyte (N:L) ratio to help in predicting prognosis (a lower ratio appears to be better for some other cancers), but this is preliminary research. The real take home point is that when some or many of the CBC numbers become severely reduced, they may need medications or even less commonly, transfusions to improve them. This is true for red blood cell indicators (Hemoglobin/Hematocrit/Red Blood Cells or RBCs), white blood cell numbers, and even the platelets, which help in blood clotting. Some treatments such as chemotherapy or radiopharmaceutical (radium-223) or radio-ligand drugs (lutetium-177) can reduce these numbers as they also eliminate cancer cells, but your medical team can give you treatments to improve those numbers if you need them. However, there is a tipping point where CBC numbers that are too low, and/or not responsive to treatment, or that do not improve greatly with treatment could then represent a change in your prognosis. For example, some men with extensive bone metastasis could see a large drop in these numbers because the cancer is impacting the blood cell production factory of the body (bone marrow) that makes many of these cells. Your medical team are experts at watching these numbers and helping you do what is needed to improve them when necessary.

PW Lifestyle Empowerment Moment

It is common to experience slight anemia from ADT because testosterone is needed to help produce some blood cells, especially the oxygen carrying red blood cells (RBCs) of the human body. This common type of ADT caused anemia is often known as "normocytic normochromic anemia." While on ADT many patients still make plenty of RBCs, which are normal in size ("normocytic") and normal in color ("normochromic") compared to when someone is not on ADT. However, the quantity of RBCs produced is usually a little bit less than normal (anemia), and often does not produce symptoms. In other words, I like to use this analogy: "the RBC producing factory (bone marrow) is often working fine on ADT., and the widgets (RBCs themselves) being made and used by the body are perfectly fine, or normal, but just a slightly lower number of widgets are being made while on ADT."

Since many men on ADT will experience normocytic normochromic anemia soon after starting ADT, and while on ADT, then the question has always been what lifestyle change or supplement will improve this situation as it could in some other specific anemic situations? In reality, this is a very different type of anemia compared to having a low iron level (microcytic anemia), or a low vitamin B12 and/or folate level (macrocytic anemia). There is no real nutrient deficiency here, but rather a purposeful testosterone deficiency. Therefore, no supplements have been proven to help this specific condition. However, there are preliminary studies of aerobic and especially resistance exercise either slightly improving this type of anemia in some men or having no impact at all. Regardless, we know exercise can improve the quality or quantity of many lives even if it is not always able to improve the quality or quantity of RBCs.

Interestingly, as we simply age there is the normal anemia of aging, especially as men make less testosterone. Also, there is anemia in some cases impacted by lifestyle, where for example excessive alcohol intake can cause a deficiency in a nutrient such as vitamin B12. There are also some medications that unknowingly could block or impact the absorption of these same nutrients such as B12 again (e.g., acid reflux drugs, metformin, etc.). In these cases, supplementation may be necessary if your medical team detects it and suggests it. Finally, excess weight gain or obesity has also been associated with lower levels of B12 and some other nutrients (including vitamin D).

14. Hormone reduction treatment choice (ADT, LHRH, newer daily antagonist pills, or surgical testicular removal)

As we discussed earlier, maintaining a castrate level of testosterone is recommended for most AdvPCa patients. But is it better to reduce testosterone by using regular LHRH/GnRH injections, newer GnRH antagonist pills, or just to have the testicles surgically removed? There has been no strong research to show that there is a survival or prognostic advantage of one method over the other. However, in some surveys of patients there seems to be a quality-of-life benefit for those who have perceived testosterone suppression flexibility or receive regular LHRH (agonist or antagonist) treatments versus a permanent testicle removal procedure. Regardless, patients receiving hormone suppressive treatment such as injections must visit their medical teams frequently to receive the injection/treatment, and that may be a positive thing.

Newer daily GnRH antagonist pills options are also now available, which preliminary encouraging evidence suggests could lower the cardiovascular risk of ADT in those with existing cardiovascular issues and provides even more choices for many patients. Taking these drugs should also encourage regular clinical visits with your medical team. Regular office visits or treatment may provide the patient and partner with a feeling of control over the process, more educational empowerment, and allow him to avoid surgery to permanently remove the testicles. Still, it is worth noting that many patients who take hormone reducing treatment by injections or other means will not start to produce testosterone at the same level again, or at all, in some cases, with years of treatment, even if the treatment is stopped. A patient who has to travel long distances and relies less on visits with the doctor may benefit from surgical removal of the testicles, but it could also be argued that increasing telehealth or facetime doctor visits allows more interactions with your medical team without having to visit in person as often. In other words, surgical testicular removal should arguably be used only in rare cases today based on patient surveys and the sheer flexibility or number of ADT options available.

15. Imaging test results over time (bone scans, MRI, PET/CT scans, etc.) & what and when you eat and exercise (lifestyle) before some scans could impact the accuracy of some of your results.

Bone scans, MRIs, PET/CT scans, PET/MRI (combination of the two), and other imaging tests can show if a cancer could be spreading to more body sites, despite being on a certain treatment, which suggests other treatment options should also now be considered. Cancer that is not spreading or tumors that are shrinking in size are both indicators that the patient could be responding to treatment. More information on imaging tests can be found throughout this book. When it comes to advances in AdvPCa, treatment medications or drugs tend to receive most of the attention. Although this is understandable, there are multiple other incredible innovations, including advances in cancer imaging taking place now.

Newer imaging tests are allowing these older and newer drugs to be used earlier when they can be more effective in many cases. Newer MRI scans can find cancer in and around the area of the prostate and potentially in nearby structures such as the seminal vesicles of neighboring lymph nodes. Newer PET/CT options, for example, can also find cancer when it is much smaller in and around the prostate, lymph nodes, bones, and other sites even further from the prostate. In general, the earlier you find advanced or advancing prostate cancer, the more likely you are to hit it with the most effective treatment(s) for your personal situation. This is very exciting!

Currently, for example, there are several different FDA approved molecules utilized with PET/CT scans that can enhance the ability to find cancer whether it is in the prostate, nodes, bones, or organs. These molecules or compounds take advantage of the fact that many cancers usually ingest or produce similar looking compounds and when this occurs with this specialized similar looking manufactured product then the location and relative size of the cancer lights up on a screen. There are PET/CT scans using FDG, which is essentially a glucose (sugar-like) molecule, being used in many different cancers, but not as often in prostate cancer, because the molecule (FDG) is not often absorbed so it does not find many prostate cancers. Still, FDG may play a role in finding some rare variants or uniquely aggressive prostate cancers that are not detected with other more commonly used prostate cancer PET/CT molecules. There is also a choline PET/CT, which can find prostate cancer within different locations in the body now being used at some select centers such as the Mayo Clinic. Additionally, there is an Axumin (fluciclovine) PET/CT, which is widely available and also FDA approved to pick up prostate cancer in some situations. Finally, there are the newer PSMA scans. In fact, PSMA PET/CT scans are the newest molecules to be used to find prostate cancer and are becoming widely available, including a special type of PSMA scan known as "Pylarify." The point here is the newer imaging advances in prostate cancer, including specialized PET/CT scans, are nothing short of amazing! Which imaging test, option, or molecule could be right for you (Axumin, Choline, FDG, PSMA, etc.) should always be discussed with your medical team.

PW Lifestyle Empowerment Moment

Diet and supplements have the potential to play an unusually important and even concerning temporary role in the future of several different PET/CT scans, such as PSMA. This is an area desperate for more awareness, so let us give it the attention it deserves. For example, many PET/CT scans discourage eating, or at least eating certain foods before the scan is completed because compounds in these foods could literally compete with the actual molecule being used in the imaging test. In other words, it could get ingested by the cancer or another location and then the similar laboratory created molecule, which helps the PET scan light up and locate the cancer, does not get absorbed. This could result in a false negative finding or a suggestion the cancer site is not as large or extensive.

Again, the created molecule in many of these imaging tests are used because they are commonly and quickly ingested or consumed by cancer cells. Cancer cells can gobble up many types of diverse molecules from amino acids (building blocks of protein), glucose (one building block of sugar), fatty acids (building blocks of fats), and numerous other compounds.

This does not suggest that eliminating these specific food sources of these molecules could stop the cancer because cancer uses so many diverse externally and internally derived (tumor produced) compounds to survive (more on this in the lifestyle section of the book). Rather, it demonstrates today how imaging tests use or take advantage of some molecules also found in diet, and for a good reason. If we know a cancer cell is more likely to quickly use a compound given by IV for example, then that same compound can be used to help medical teams find precisely where your cancer is located.

It is for this reason there are PET/CT scans using manufactured compounds that look similar to glucose molecules (FDG-PET/CT scan), amino acid compounds (Axumin/fluciclovine scan), fatty acids or essential nutrient building blocks of cell membranes (choline scan). Again, most of these compounds are identical, or at least somewhat similar in structure to what is found in some of our diets! Wow! The manufactured food-like molecules utilized in these scans help the scan "light up," so you can see where the cancer exists.

However, what if you were to eat this same molecule in food around the time of the scan? Could it theoretically reduce the ability to see cancer or tumors because it would be taken up by the cancer cells and compete with the manufactured molecular product, which has been specifically designed to light up when ingested by cancer, which is given to you before your scan? For example, the choline PET/CT scan, which again is used in the U.S. today at some distinguished medical centers such as the Mayo Clinic, has beautifully and accurately written within the prescribing rules and patient instructions the following: "Fasting for at least six hours is recommended to minimize the potential for dietary choline interference with radioactivity uptake in tissues." Research is looking at all these questions right now. In the meantime, companies are trying to adjust to this potential interference with scans research. Another example is the latest patient handout from the company providing the Axumin scan which wonderfully states "to avoid any significant exercise for at least a full 24 hours prior to your Axumin PET/CT scan." Additionally, it states "Do not eat or drink for at least 4 hours prior to your PET/CT scan (other than small amounts of water for taking medications)."

However, what appears to be currently overlooked, in general, in this research are all the dietary supplements and countless other products that contain compounds that could theoretically interfere with the uptake of the manufactured compounds used for PET/CT scans. For example, products with choline, glucose, or even those with the compound glutamine or glutamate (compounds which are somewhat similar to the structure of the PSMA molecule). In fact, today there are numerous over the counter products, and even prescription medicines, that contain large amounts of these substances. What about those? Shouldn't they also be temporarily (not permanently) restricted for some time right before one of these scans is performed? I believe it needs to be considered based on the latest data, but at the very least this issue needs to be discussed. So, again, please ask your medical team about the very latest and greatest research in this area of diet, supplements, or other pills and lifestyle changes (exercise, etc.).

For example, right before this book was published new research suggested some COVID-19 vaccines could cause temporary lymph node enlargement near the site of injection after the first dose is given and an even higher number of individuals experience this impact after the second injection for at least several weeks. This is known for example by the name "vaccine-induced axillary lymphadenopathy." The good news is that this temporary lymph node enlargement does not appear to occur in most patients within the first few weeks of receiving the vaccine, but still, it is not a small percentage (perhaps up to 25% of patients could experience it in some studies). Temporary lymph node enlargement from a vaccine is not a concern unless someone gets a PET/CT scan and their recent vaccine use is not known, which could theoretically cause a health care professional to think it is a potential site of cancer rather than a temporary enlargement of a lymph node caused by a recent preventive (COVID-19 for example) vaccine.

The lesson here is health care professionals and patients should have a discussion not only about diet and exercise before a scan but what vaccines, if any, were received recently or could be delayed a few weeks before receiving some scans. All these newer impacts of lifestyle behaviors on scans are fascinating and simultaneously concerning if not known, and thus need to be updated and better known. Interestingly, there have been past and current examples of what you eat or do impacting your imaging results. For example, some medical centers (not all) want you to consume a low-residue or low intestinal gas producing diet (aka low in fiber or fiber restricted), or potentially a liquid-based diet a day (length varies per center) before an MRI thus minimizing gas produced in the intestines during the scan because it could obscure or interfere with the pictures or readings. Some centers also suggest avoiding sexual activity approximately three or more days before a prostate MRI scan to enhance the reading of some of the areas of the prostate itself and/or adjacent to the prostate for example, such as the seminal vesicles (SV), because this tissue area could temporarily decrease in size after ejaculation and reduce the resolution of this area of the body. In other words, the SV volumes are larger in some men if they abstain from ejaculation for at least three days and this could partially enhance or improve the accuracy of the scan.

Additionally, the bone scan has been around for a long time, and it is now appreciated that if compounds or commercial products with bismuth in them (such as Pepto-Bismol, generic equivalents, etc.) are ingested within several days of this scan and possibly other imaging tests (X-ray, CT, etc.) then the bismuth could light up in some cases on the scan making it look like something concerning is there in that body location where it is being digested when in reality it is not concerning—it is just Pepto-Bismol (note: bismuth is what is known as a "radiopaque" substance). I believe there is so much more to be learned! "Lifestyle changes can change so many aspects of life!" I apologize, but I had to use another one of my favorite quotations.

16. Lactate/Lactic Acid Dehydrogenase (LDH) blood test

Lactate/lactic acid dehydrogenase is an important enzyme found in most tissues of the body. It can be measured in a blood test and help to predict the aggressiveness of your AdvPCa, or what the cancer could be doing right now. An abnormally high level of this enzyme tends to suggest an increase in cellular injury and that the cancer could be acting more aggressively in the body. On the other hand, a reduction in this number could indicate a positive response to treatment.

17. Mental health (stress, anxiety, depression and associated conditions or issues)

There has been considerable controversy over the impact of mental health on a cancer prognosis. When mental health is not optimal, it can certainly impact physical health and vice versa. Additionally, cancer can increase the risk of mental health issues and has been shown to potentially make existing issues even worse, unless treated properly. Stress, anxiety, depression (I like to call it the "S.A.D." acronym for simplicity, emphasis, and increased awareness, so that it is remembered and discussed as much as physical health) should be addressed regularly by every patient, partner, and their medical team. Stress, anxiety, and depression can cause delays in treatment, as well as make side effects from treatment worse, thus negatively impacting prognosis in some cases. Also, even when cancer treatments are working well, when these mental health issues are not addressed or treated, it becomes more difficult to feel like you are winning the battle against cancer. The good news is there are many interventions, including in-person or telemedicine therapy, lifestyle changes, medications, and support groups. So, be sure to include how you are coping mentally before, during or after any cancer treatment in discussions with your healthcare team. Unfortunately, the lack of awareness of options is still a problem. Mental health is arguably one of the least appreciated parts of the prognosis puzzle, but you and your medical team have the power to immediately change this statistic, so please never hesitate to talk to your team about any of these issues.

PW Lifestyle Empowerment Moment

It is tough to appreciate the research that suggests that even when someone is being treated for mental health issues with medications and other conventional treatments, lifestyle changes, such as exercise or socialized exercise (working out with a group, or another person, trainer, or in a social setting) has only further improved the response to treatment in many individuals. Conventional treatment and exercise could also be helpful for patients prone to S.A.D., or related conditions such as "catastrophizing," which is dealing with persistent or regular negative beliefs in assuming the worst-case scenario will usually occur despite evidence to the contrary. It is a persistent, pervasive and at times debilitating type of negative thinking, which can be associated with many mental health situations including stress, anxiety or depression. There has also been a great deal of research on the mental health detriments of cancer treatment, especially ADT lately, but again the impact of daily or regular exercise in reducing these cognitive risks cannot be overemphasized.

Finally, please remember the name "HIPPOCAMPUS," because it is found in each temporal lobe (left and right) of the brain, and recent research suggests it is highly sensitive to physical activity. It not only increases blood flow to this area, but also stimulates the delivery of compounds within it, and to it. Therefore, exercise helps improve or maintain hippocampal size and function, whether you are 21 or 101 years of age. It is part of the reason the brain is also now considered a "use it or lose it" organ. Why is the hippocampus so special? The hippocampus is one of the primary areas of the brain involved in memory. It may even be a partial explanation why the American Academy of Neurology (AAN) recently changed their clinical guidelines to include exercise as a potential way of preventing mild cognitive impairment (MCI) from becoming dementia, and this was based on past clinical research. Please prescribe, recommend, or simply exercise regularly for better overall mental health wellness, especially when dealing with the hormonal changes of prostate cancer treatment, which has also been associated with cognitive issues. In other words, please make exercise a mental health wellness rule and not an exception, and you and your medical team will FEEL the empowerment of this lifestyle change!

18. Pain

Men with AdvPCa and varying pain levels tend to have different prognoses. The worse the pain or symptoms caused by the cancer itself, the worse the prognosis or the more serious the situation. This makes sense because tumors that have grown large enough to cause pain are more troubling than smaller tumors not causing pain. Similarly, the more pain control or medication needed because of an advanced symptomatic cancer then the more likely the cancer has become more aggressive. Pain control is critical and is absolutely necessary, but it also gives a glimpse of what could be going on inside the body. Pain caused by other chronic conditions, such as arthritis, does not play a role in this consideration. However, other reasons for non-cancerous pain or discomfort also need attention because it impacts mental health and overall quality of life.

19. Partner/life partner/support network (it is a Couple's Disease)

Approximately 30 years ago when I began writing my first prostate cancer book, I remember mentioning preliminary studies suggesting a potential survival advantage for men with prostate cancer that also had a life partner or were in a close relationship versus men not in a strong relationship. Thus, whether an association or causation, as we say, there are known quality of life benefits to having people in your life to support you through this journey. Support groups (virtual or in-person) and advocacy groups have also become a wonderful source of information. Now, I do not think there will be a definitive major study to settle the verdict on the impact of prognosis when receiving support, but personally I believe there is an advantage mentally, which could translate to a physical and survival advantage for some men. I also believe there is an informational advantage to having a partner or support group that could open more doors to treatment options and experiences.

Still, I should add one note of caution, because I also remember 30 years ago preliminary research from major medical centers throughout the world that demonstrated the impact of cancer on the partner of the man going through prostate cancer treatment. It appeared the mental health impact on the partner without cancer was indeed similar to the patient with cancer! Today, this is not as much of a surprise based on recent research, but it is still not recognized enough. Prostate cancer is a COUPLE'S DISEASE or even a family's disease in many cases, and it should be treated this way by the couple themselves, family, and their medical team. Both individuals going through the experience must make each other the primary priority, during the good and the challenging times. Okay, sorry, I will get off my soapbox now, but coming from a family filled with cancer, I have seen the importance of this evidence-based advice over and over again.

20. Performance status (ECOG, etc.) or scale

Performance status is a scale that attempts to quantify or grade the general well-being or quality of life of a patient. Healthcare professionals use the scale to determine whether someone should receive treatment, whether a dosage change is needed, or if therapy should even be continued for a particular patient. Two commonly used scales are the Eastern Cooperative Oncology Group (ECOG), which is one of the largest and most respected clinical cancer research organizations, and the Karnofsky Performance Scale or Status, which was named for Dr. David A. Karnofsky, an oncologist dedicated to treating cancer patients and ensuring quality-of-life measures be appreciated when undergoing treatment. A brief description of each of the two scales follows. Overall, a poor performance status indicates a worse prognosis as compared to someone with a better performance status.

Numerous drug clinical trials require an ECOG performance status of 0 to 2 to be allowed to participate in them. There are exceptions, but often patients with scores of 3 or 4 have more difficulty qualifying for some treatments, or the standard dosage and/or frequency of treatments, because the possibility of the benefit is outweighed by the potential of serious negative side effects. Again, each case is different, and there are exceptions. This should be a discussion between you and your partner and your medical team. It is also critical to mention that performance status is just a snapshot of one point in your journey, and it can change in both directions—not just progress to worse numbers, but with good responses to today's treatments it could also result in better prognostic or lower ECOG numbers or higher Karnofsky scores.

ECOG Performance Status or Grade

In general, the *lower* the number the better the prognosis or situation.

ECOG Score of 0 = Asymptomatic (fully active, no restrictions)
ECOG Score of 1 = Symptomatic and fully able to walk (can perform light work, such as household or office tasks, but cannot do strenuous activities)
ECOG Score of 2 = Symptomatic and spends less than 50% of time in bed (can walk and provide self-care, but unable to do work activities)
ECOG Score of 3 = Symptomatic and spends more than 50% of time in bed or chair (not bedbound, capable of limited self-care)
ECOG Score of 4 = Bedbound (cannot provide for self-care, completely confined to bed or chair)

Karnofsky Performance Status (KPS) Scale or Grade

In general, the higher the number the better the prognosis or situation. KPS can be expressed as a range (90-100) or a specific number (92 for example).

100 = Normal, no complaints or signs of disease
90 = Normal activity, few symptoms or signs of disease
80 = Normal activity, some symptoms or signs of disease
70 = Caring for self, not capable of normal activity or work
60 = Needs some help, can take care of personal requirements
50 = Needs help often, requires frequent medical care
40 = Disabled, needs special help and care
30 = Severely disabled, hospital admission indicated but no danger of death
20 = Very ill, urgently needing admission and supportive measures of treatment
10 = Rapidly progressive

Thus, an ECOG score of 0 is approximately similar to a KPS of 90-100, and an ECOG of 1 is similar to a KPS of 70-80s, and so on.

21. Preventive vaccines (vaccine preventable illnesses) for adults, including COVID-19

Adult preventive vaccination compliance is approximately 25-50% in general. This is a big problem in adults for many reasons. For example, pneumonia is still a top cause of morbidity and mortality, and shingles can not only cause debilitating nerve pain (post-herpetic neuralgia or PHN) that could last for months to years, but if shingles gets into the eyes (known as HZO or Herpes Zoster Ophthalmicus) it can cause (or exacerbate) glaucoma, cataracts, or temporary and even permanent vision loss. Furthermore, and perhaps even more surprising, shingles is associated with an increased risk of some cardiovascular events, including stroke, because it can cause tremendous inflammation and blockage of important blood vessels. Interestingly, many other vaccine preventable illnesses are also associated with an increase in cardiovascular events. COVID-19 is now known to also increase the risk of such events, so it would not be surprising if this newer vaccination is ultimately demonstrated to reduce the risk of some of these cardiovascular issues. Preliminary evidence suggests several different viruses including the one causing shingles could temporarily increase PSA levels in the body in very rare situations. Regardless, the take home point here is critical—please talk to your medical team to see which adult vaccines you need right now, or in the future, so this critically important area of your health is not overlooked. Many of these vaccine preventable illnesses such as COVID-19, shingles, and pneumonia could cause major delays in your cancer treatment, as well as increase the risk of many health problems. Adult vaccinations should receive more attention for their potential diverse side benefits compared to their side effects.

> ### *PW Lifestyle Empowerment Moment*
>
> Recent evidence from Medicare and other databases suggests the shingles vaccination is associated with a reduction in cardiovascular events. Interestingly, the newest shingles vaccine (Shingrix) utilizes an adjuvant (something to boost the immune response of the product) from the Soap Bark Tree in Chile, so it could

even be considered a nature-derived vaccine. One of the COVID-19 prevention vaccines also utilizes an adjuvant from the Soap Bark Tree. Furthermore, the side benefits of other vaccines are receiving clinical trials right now, such as the tetanus shot being used to enhance the dendritic cell immunotherapy treatment against certain brain tumors. Finally, past and recent research continues to suggest heart healthy behaviors could be associated with greater immunological responses (higher antibody titers), or improved protection after receiving some common preventive vaccines (e.g., hepatitis, influenza, pneumonia, etc.). In other words, lifestyle factors such as maintaining a healthy weight, diet, exercise, better sleep quality and/or quantity, and others that we are emphasizing in the book appear to be immune healthy. Heart Healthy=Immune Healthy! It is time to consider many of these vaccine preventable illnesses as not only being infectious diseases but cardiovascular diseases. By preventing them with vaccines the side benefits could translate into diverse quality and quantity of life benefits!

22. Previous responses to treatment(s) and/or how well you are able to tolerate treatment(s) after they have been initiated.

Response to previous prostate cancer, or just AdvPCa treatment, is a good indicator of prognosis or the aggressiveness of your tumor. For example, someone who responded well to several cycles of chemotherapy, or an androgen receptor inhibitor (ARI) pill has a better prognosis compared to someone who only responded for a short time or not at all. Positive responses to one or more treatments for AdvPCa is a good indicator that this same individual could respond favorably to other treatments. In addition, the ability to tolerate treatment so you can continue to receive uninterrupted treatment is another part of this prognostic indicator that does not receive enough attention. If someone is healthier, or more fit, and able to tolerate treatment then they are less likely to experience major delays in their treatment. So, it is not only the health or performance status of the patient starting treatment (ECOG status), but how well they do after experiencing some of the side effects of these many AdvPCa options. Today, there are so many treatment options, but being able to use them at the precise time they are needed is critical. In other words, using my favorite athletic analogy, the more times you get up to bat then the more likely you are to swing and hit a single, double, triple, homerun, or grand slam. Another reason why diverse sources of educational empowerment, put into action, are so powerful!

23. Primary tumor site status and treatment, debulking, or "local control" of an advanced cancer

This used to be a controversial prognostic indicator, but today there is enough research to suggest it could make a difference for some patients and should be discussed with your medical team. In some other tumor types, such as colon, kidney, and ovarian, a person with advanced cancer may have a better prognosis when the primary tumor, or the location where the tumor initially began to grow is treated with radiation or removed (debulked). It appears that treating the part of the body where the tumor started growing, and continues to grow, despite the cancer spreading far beyond these areas could still provide a benefit. How? Simply radiating, removing, or treating the primary tumor may make it less able to send out more cancer cells into the rest of the body, or even communicate with other tumor cells in the body. Does this mean that men with AdvPCa should get radiation to the prostate (first or second time, etc.), or have it removed or treated? Again, there are now some preliminary clinical studies suggesting a potential benefit, which is also known as "local control" of an advanced cancer especially when the disease is not as widespread within the body. Still, discussing whether you are a candidate for debulking, or "cytoreductive" treatment, or localized control despite having advanced disease (advantages and disadvantages) should occur with your medical team. This will be an ongoing area of controversy, research and continued interest because as better treatments continue to be approved it could reduce, enhance, or even have no impact on the efficacy of this approach.

24. PSA and PSA Kinetics (PSADT—PSA Doubling Time or PSAV—PSA Velocity, stable PSA, % changes or reductions in PSA, etc.)

Increasing PSA, rapidly increasing PSA or doubling time (i.e., the PSA doubles every 3-12 months vs 2-3 years) could all be indicators of a worse prognosis. Conversely, the longer it takes PSA to double during treatment the more likely this is a favorable prognostic sign as are stabilizations or even percentage drops in PSA (>50%, 50%, 33%, 25%, etc.). But keep in mind there are exceptions to this rule. For example, Provenge or Xofigo treatment for AdvPCa does not consistently impact or reduce PSA levels, but these treatments are associated with a better survival rate. On the other hand, chemotherapy (Taxotere, Jevtana, etc.) tends to lower PSA or slow the rise in PSA in many men, and it is also associated with an improved survival rate for AdvPCa. There are also rare cases where very aggressive tumors don't produce PSA and where less aggressive tumors create a lot of PSA. In fact, some men diagnosed with PSA levels in the 1000s have amazing initial responses to treatment despite these very large PSA numbers. Yet, this also reflects a prostate cancer with an ability to still produce a lot of PSA or still having the normal machinery inside the cell to make PSA, which suggests it would respond to treatment. This contrasts with the man with a very low PSA at diagnosis, but with cancer throughout the body. This is observed in some rare cases of very aggressive tumors that no longer act normally, and do not even contain the normal machinery to make much PSA because it is acting so abnormally or aggressive (i.e., very different from a traditional prostate cancer). In these rare cases, your medical team has other options including imaging and even other blood tests (ALP, D-Dimer, Fibrinogen, LDH, etc.) to determine if the cancer is progressing despite a stable (non-moving PSA). Still, PSA levels and kinetics are very informative, which is part of the reason PSA is arguably the most reliable or best cancer blood test ever invented after someone has been diagnosed and treated for prostate cancer. The take home message—PSA and PSA kinetics, along with the location of the tumor(s) in the body are important discussions before, during, and after any treatment.

25. Sarcopenia Severity (quality, quantity, and function)— the new prostate cancer epidemic? Yes!

"Sarco" means flesh and "-penia" means lack of, and loss of muscle quantity, quality and/or function (i.e., strength, coordination, balance). Sarcopenia, which is the loss of muscle mass related to aging and/or immobility, is one of the most underappreciated side effects and prognostic indicators of cancer treatment. However, this is changing and now there is enormous attention being placed on this diagnosis or condition. It has become common for men on ADT/AdvPCa to experience some type of sarcopenia because of a lack of testosterone, which helps maintain or improve muscle quantity, quality and function, along with impacting many other factors, such as energy levels. The muscles are a "use it or lose it" group of tissues that have nerves and blood vessels running through them and they also help support many of the bones and joints throughout the body. Greater losses of muscle mass, quality and function from cancer, or even as a side effect from ADT or other treatments, makes it harder to handle treatment itself, fight cancer, and simply maintain a good quality of life. Greater muscle quantity and quality is associated with better metabolism, higher energy levels, and arguably a host of other beneficial qualities that give someone the extra strength needed to handle treatment, as well as activities of daily living (ADL). If you have experienced noticeable loss of muscle strength and/or size, or function then please discuss this with your healthcare team.

PW Lifestyle Empowerment Moment

I find it interesting that no major medications have been discovered with ADT/AdvPCa that work as well as exercise to prevent sarcopenia in cancer patients. In other words, exercise, not just aerobic or flexibility exercises, but also resistance exercise (some type of regular light weightlifting, use of resistance bands, or using different body positions or poses as resistance exercise) should be mandatory when approved by your medical team, and it should be regularly discussed with your medical team.

In my mind PSA should also mean "Preventing Sarcopenia with Aging" because it is that important. Sarcopenia prevention also supports balance and prevents bone loss, which then reduces the risk of falls and fractures in men and women. It could be the difference between tolerating treatment or not, as well as preventing delays in your treatment. In addition, the mental health benefits of exercise are so potentially amazing that everyone that is approved from their medical team to do any form of exercise should be out there exercising regularly or even daily. Please do this! Thank you.

26. Spiritual health

Most medical teams inquire about individual spiritual beliefs or customs, and they passionately honor them. In general, studies suggest individuals committed to some form of spiritual health appear to have an improved quality of life. But why? Is it because it's associated with more positive thinking or optimism? Is it because it's associated with a larger support network and less isolated or insular behaviors? Is it because of a higher power? Could quantity of life be impacted by spirituality? These debates or discussions will always be a part of the research. I never thought it was my role to wax personal spiritual beliefs in this book, but rather to report the research (good and bad). With that being said, there is sufficient supportive evidence, although preliminary, that a commitment to something, or some cause greater than self, appears to be associated with an improvement in self. This is part of the potential intrinsic beauty within the spiritual health research. Objectively speaking, it is inclusive, diverse, and the true meaning of spirituality from the research provides for plenty of latitude, as is should. People find belief, worship, or their personal sense of spirituality in many different formats, communities, or avenues, and yet we are all still linked by something inherently beautiful. Whether or not your spiritual beliefs are important to you is yet another important subject your medical team would be honored to know.

27. Stage of Cancer ("How far it has spread in the body")

Staging is a system used to identify where a cancer is located and how far it has spread. The TNM staging system is the most common one used for prostate cancer. The acronym stands for primary tumor location (T), lymph nodes (N), and metastases (M). The tumor location is based on the results of a clinical examination, imaging tests, a biopsy, and blood tests. The node assessment is generally based on a clinical examination, imaging, or lymph node removal. The assessment of metastases uses clinical examination, imaging, specific bone or skeletal studies, and blood tests. Every prostate cancer should ideally be given a T, N, and M assessment. An "x" or "0" score for the T, N, or M indicator usually means that either the location of the tumor cannot be determined currently (e.g., Tx, Nx, or Mx) or there is no evidence of cancer in that area after evaluation (e.g., T0, N0, or M0, 0 meaning "zero"). Subcategories can be used to provide a more exact tumor location, but those subcategories won't be covered here because in treating AdvPCa patients more emphasis is placed on the N and M staging. This is because the cancer is often advanced to that point (i.e., regional or non-regional lymph nodes, bones, etc.). Patients with a higher or greater TNM stage or number and/or letter have a more concerning prognosis than patients with a lower TNM stage or number and/or letter. Again, if someone has a good or great response to treatment then things could change for the better quickly and they may be more favorably restaged because some tumor sites are no longer visible. This has happened to some patients being treated with both older and newer medications.

28. Time from Initial Treatment to AdvPCa Diagnosis, or Time on ADT before progressing (converting) to CRPC

If you were treated for localized prostate cancer, and then it rapidly progressed to become advanced or even AdvPCa, this could indicate a more aggressive cancer. However, if you were diagnosed and treated for localized prostate cancer, and many years later the disease came back, and several or many

Primary Tumor Location (T stage)	What does this mean?
T1	Tumor is within the prostate and found only by PSA and biopsy alone, or using another non-cancer prostate procedure (for example TURP), but was not found by imaging or digital rectal exam.
T2	Tumor is within the prostate and found by digital rectal exam, combined digital rectal exam and PSA testing, imaging, or from localized treatment.
T3	Tumor has grown through the prostate capsule (tissue that surrounds the prostate itself) and/or into the seminal vesicles.
T4	Tumor has spread further to areas adjacent to or near the prostate, such as the bladder neck, external sphincter, levator muscles, pelvic wall, or rectum.

Regional Lymph Nodes (nodes near the prostate or within the pelvic area, N stage)	What does this mean?
Nx	Regional lymph nodes cannot be evaluated right now.
N0	No regional lymph nodes have cancer.
N1	Regional lymph node(s) has some cancer.

Metastatic Disease (M stage)	What does this mean?
Mx or determined right now.	Distant metastases could not be evaluated
M0	No distant metastases.
M1a	Non-regional (beyond the pelvic area) lymph node(s) have some cancer; either side or both sides of the body are involved.
M1b	Cancer has spread to the bone(s).
M1c	Cancer has spread to other sites or organs in the body (for example, lung or liver).

years after that it became AdvPCa, it would imply a slower, or steadier cancer that may have a better prognosis. Similarly, the shorter the time it takes to go from a more localized disease in and around the prostate, to being diagnosed with one or more bone metastasis then the more aggressive the cancer, whereas the longer it takes for the cancer to move to the bones the potentially less aggressive the cancer. Another way to look at this, which is receiving more attention now, is the shorter the time you were on ADT before progressing or becoming CRPC then the more aggressive the cancer for many (not all) men. For example, if you were placed on ADT before being diagnosed with CRPC and it took less than one year to progress to CRPC, versus 3 years, then the man with the shorter initial time to CRPC conversion (one year) would be expected to have a more aggressive prostate cancer.

29. Total Testosterone (TT) Levels before ADT

There is some preliminary controversial but also interesting research to suggest that a patient who had an abnormally low testosterone level before receiving treatment for AdvPCa could have a more aggressive prostate cancer compared to someone with a more normal level for their age. This is preliminary but makes some sense: If a cancer was growing or can grow with less testosterone (fuel for many prostate cancers) for some time, then giving ADT could be less effective since a partial androgen suppressive situation was already occurring in the body. In other words, some of these prostate cancer cells may have already found a way to survive without much testosterone around. Regardless, the take home message here is knowing your total testosterone level before being treated with ADT/AdvPCa could provide some potential insight for some men and their medical team.

PW Lifestyle Empowerment Moment

Why does obesity result in more aggressive tumors in some men, or less response to ADT in other men? Is it because obese men on average have significantly lower levels of testosterone compared to similar aged men of lesser weight or waist size? Testosterone enhancing drugs when given to a man with prostate cancer could provide fuel for tumors to grow larger and faster. This is why taking testosterone enhancing supplements are also so concerning when dealing with prostate cancer. The potential exception to this rule is within metastatic CRPC (mCRPC), which is currently being studied in clinical trials and discussed later in the book. This is known as bipolar androgen therapy or BAT or rapid cycling high testosterone therapy, and though interesting, it's still experimental. The idea in clinical trials right now is to continue to be on ADT, but also add testosterone injections every 28 days or so in an attempt to sensitize/re-sensitize CRPC to an anti-androgen treatment, such as an androgen-receptor inhibitor (ARI), after a patient no longer responds to another anti-androgen treatment. You can check with your medical team about the status of this research (good or bad).

On a separate lifestyle note, as men without prostate cancer have spent billions of dollars on testosterone replacement therapy (TRT) over the past decade there is something getting missed in the excitement to use these drugs. One of the greatest testosterone reducers in an adult man of any age is weight or waist gain, and recent clinical studies are showing that as men lose weight, or waist, testosterone can increase in some cases without the need for TRT. Now, a testosterone increase does not occur on ADT with weight loss, in general, because the drug is usually too strong to allow it. ADT itself encourages further weight and waist gain, but men on ADT that are able to maintain their weight or waist tend to feel better.

Interestingly, it is not well-known that in some areas of the world the monthly ADT injection dosage is half, or 50% less, but still just as effective. Why? In these areas of the world, the average patient is smaller, or harbors less weight and waist and lower BMI (on average), so the body is arguably more sensitive to this specific drug in these cases, compared to a person of higher body weight or waist. In other words, less drug is required, and this is also the case today with some chemotherapy drugs throughout the world, where part of the dosage given is based on weight. Other drugs are less weight based. Still, the take home message is that ADT encourages weight and waist increases of primarily subcutaneous (right under the skin), and visceral (deeper inside the body around organs) adipose/fat tissue. Thus, preventing substantial weight gain on ADT is extremely difficult and needs to be supported to improve quality of life and reduce the multiple and diverse potential side effects of ADT. In fact, some past and recent research on hot flashes suggest that heavier individuals experience more hot flashes when starting ADT and/or may have a greater number of severe hot flashes. This phenomenon has also been observed in breast cancer patients using hormone reducing therapies.

30. Visceral or soft-tissue disease

The literal meaning of visceral is "of the internal organs" and this has come to mean cancer that has spread to locations apart from the prostate or bones, such as the liver, lungs, or other areas well beyond the prostate. Individuals who have visceral disease or cancer in multiple areas of the body and around the prostate (or where the prostate used to be located in some cases) have a more challenging prognosis than those without disease in these areas. This is because the disease has advanced further. In fact, the actual organ of metastasis itself may also be more immediately concerning versus other areas. For example, a liver or lung metastasis may suggest more aggressive cancer compared to cancer in a different organ or part of the body. The situation is similar to what is called "soft-tissue disease," where the cancer has spread to non-bony areas such as organs and/or regional or non-regional lymph nodes. The further a cancer has traveled beyond the regional lymph nodes, which are near the

Pelvic Nodes

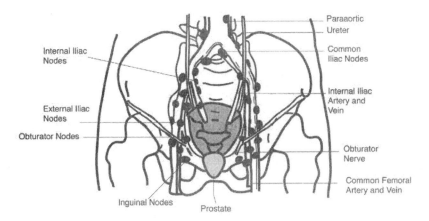

The pelvic lymph nodes are the first set of nodes in the human body where prostate cancer usually goes after growing beyond the prostate area.

Abdominal Nodes

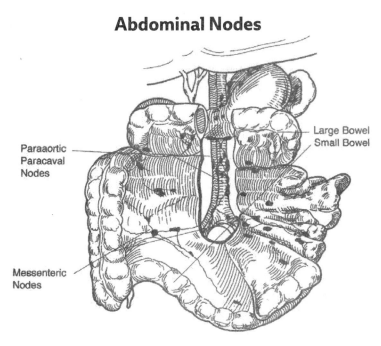

The abdominal pelvic lymph nodes are the second set of nodes where cancer may typically spread.

Peri Hilar/Supraclavicular Nodes

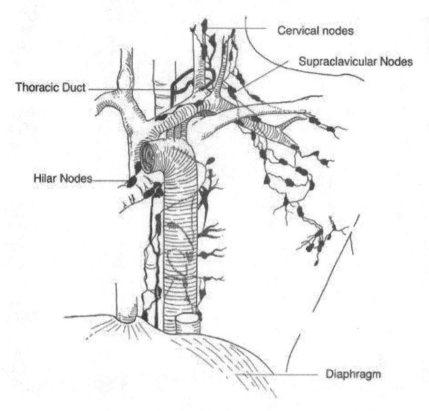

The Peri Hilar/Supraclavicular lymph nodes, located generally speaking in the chest and neck area, are usually the third set of nodes where prostate cancer spreads.

prostate, or more distant areas (non-regional nodes) then the further advanced and more concerning the prostate cancer (see also "Staging" in this chapter).

What has been harder to appreciate is the somewhat organized progressive movement of prostate cancer from the prostate itself to the rest of the body, when the cancer is aggressive or on the move, or not stopped by a current treatment. Prostate cancer usually spreads outward first to areas right next to the prostate (or where the prostate was) and then to the local or regional lymph nodes near the prostate, then to lymph nodes further away (non-regional lymph nodes), then to bone and finally to organs or other tissues. This is reflected in the well-researched staging system (TNM) mentioned earlier, but we decided to also show the progressive lymph node chains impacted over time. This is necessary to show or visualize the progressive and somewhat anatomically organized movement in most men (unless treated) because throughout our careers there has been a false sense of cancer simply "jumping" from the prostate right into a bone or organ—skipping part of the anatomical path along the way toward these sites. In reality, prostate cancer moves from point-to-point in the body, and if at any of those points you block its ability to keep moving forward, and/or eliminate some of the cancer at the front of the line, so to speak, then this could have a positive impact on survival. The treatments highlighted in this book, which were FDA approved because they improved survival from a phase 3 clinical trial, also have that ability to discourage the movement, pace, or progression of prostate cancer.

31. Volume (amount of Cancer) and quantity/number of sites with cancer—"oligometastatic prostate cancer (OMPC)" revisited

In general, the greater the amount of cancer in your body, the more concerning the tumor(s), and the more serious the situation. For example, someone with cancer in the lymph nodes, in some organs, and in many bones tends to have a more aggressive cancer as compared to someone with just a few tumors located on a single bone. The lower the number of metastatic spots, and/or the more concentrated they are to one area then the better the potential prognosis, which has also led to an almost universally accepted new term in prostate cancer known as "oligometastatic prostate cancer (OMPC)," which was mentioned earlier in the chapter. In general, OMPC suggests the earlier and the lower the number of metastatic sites or spots found then the better the ability to treat them. It has been variably defined by 5, 4, or even less (oligo means "few") total metastatic sites in the lymph nodes and/or bone. There is also a remarkable preliminary finding suggesting OMPC could in some cases represent a less aggressive variant of prostate cancer where in some cases just the OMPC sites are treated by radiation before giving ADT or when needing ADT. Even if diagnosed with CRPC those sites could be more responsive to treatment. Regardless, the take home message is the lower the amount of cancer (lower the volume) and/or areas of cancerous sites, and the more concentrated the better the potential prognosis, compared to someone with large amounts of cancer (higher volume), more metastatic sites, and in many different locations (not concentrated to an area). This is also why working with your medical team to find the location of your tumor sites as early as possible is an important tool in planning treatment.

32. Weight Loss (excessive/extreme) or the inability to gain weight when needed

When the cancer itself is impacting other areas of the body and causing extreme unintentional weight loss (sometimes called "cachexia"), then this usually means that the cancer has become more aggressive and occupies more of the body as compared to someone without unintentional extreme weight loss. In general, when men have minimal-to-no testosterone because of ADT/AdvPCa, there is usually some weight/waist gain because metabolism slows down dramatically, and it becomes much easier to put on weight, which is another reason why extreme unintentional weight loss is concerning. However, there could be multiple other reasons for weight loss that could not necessarily reflect prognosis, but rather an effect or side effect of a treatment. For example, some drugs may reduce appetite, cause diarrhea or nausea, or fatigue, which could lead to weight loss. If your weight has increased or decreased moderately or dramatically then it is time to talk to your healthcare team about your options.

PW Lifestyle Empowerment Moment

It is far more common to gain weight while on ADT, but there are circumstances when not only the cancer, but some prostate cancer treatments or side effects can cause weight loss. There are many potential causes for weight loss, including diarrhea, constipation, lack of appetite, nausea, pain, inflammation in or around the mouth, taste/smell changes, mental health issues, and more. It could also be due to another medication or pill not related to cancer treatment. If the weight loss is extreme enough to be compromising quality of life and the ability to continue treatment, then there are multiple options. However, the first step is addressing and treating the primary cause(s) of the weight loss. This involves a discussion about your concerns with your medical team. Some common discussions involve the use of marijuana, or even cannabis-related drug derivatives available as a prescription. One of the biggest problems in obtaining marijuana or cannabinoid compounds from less reliable sources is simply the problem of a COA, which is a "certificate of analysis" proving the product you are purchasing actually contains what is advertised (not higher or lower in dose), without additional exposure to contaminants, such as heavy metals, bacteria, fungus, herbicides, pesticides, etc. Can the company selling the product prove it's "clean?" Please make sure the product being recommended has a COA or simply comes from a reputable source.

Another popular controversial method of increasing caloric consumption comes from a variety of protein-based beverages, which now offer low, medium, and high caloric options. The good news is the taste of these products is getting better (emphasis on "getting"). However, keep in mind that one of the primary high caloric ingredients in many of these beverages is some form of concentrated plant oil(s), where one tablespoon is equivalent to 120-130 calories (primarily concentrated calories from fat), or almost the same total caloric intake of one can of sugar-sweetened soda pop. In other words, would it be cheaper, or make as much sense to just use separate tablespoons of plant oil with certain meals? The problem again would be a bland or not so exciting taste, and whether this is the real reason for the weight loss, or is this really needed or wanted. The advantage of these protein-based drinks is not only the calories, but the convenience. For someone not able to chew, sit for a meal, or digest food appropriately, then a straw and a liquid beverage is a good option. What is desperately needed in the research is a strong study of using less of these oils and sugars and healthier whole, mashed, soft, or even healthier liquid foods (i.e., veggie and/or some fruit smoothies) with protein powders added as needed, that could be more palatable for some patients losing weight. However, it is tough to get such a large study funded. In the meantime, you and your partner and healthcare team should decide what is best for you in terms of increasing your caloric intake if needed. Keep in mind, there has also been a controversial push to put weight on some people who are not able to gain weight because of the dramatic increase in metabolism (actually "catabolism") caused by the cancer itself in some cases (not because they are eating less), and to give some specific prescription options to further stimulate appetite or weight gain (such as progesterone options), and this has resulted in even further controversies. Some of these medications just increase the amount of adipose or fat tissue (not muscle quantity or quality), could increase side effects, and have had questionable quality of life benefits. In other words, if you are losing considerable amounts of weight, again first talk with your healthcare team about your eating concerns, and then determine the right path for you.

33. You and Your Medical Team Part A. Bi-directional or symbiotic relationship is as important as it gets.

Confidence in, and support from your medical team is essential. You want a team with a positive attitude and optimism, but not with exaggerated optimism or unnecessary negativity.

Multiple studies continue to find many patients with cancer, and especially advanced cancer, had minimal knowledge of their true prognosis or situation. Why? Is it because they did not want to know their prognosis if it involves bad news? Is it because some medical teams do not want to give bad news even when the situation is bad, or simply want to keep believing hopeful things will change in terms of prognosis? Regardless of the many potential reasons, part of the truth in your individualized prognosis is finding a medical team you honor, who also honors you, with honesty, sensitivity, sincerity, and hope—and never dismissive of your or your partner's thoughts and feelings. No book, no speech, no words, can give enough credibility and beauty to a patient and partner who have found the ideal medical team(s) for them, and whose medical team is simply excited, humbled, and honored by the trust you have placed in them. It is our sincere hope that you are able to find your "dream team" to help you during the good and bad times.

PW Lifestyle Empowerment Moment

There always seems to be some debate on whether a positive attitude in a patient could improve prognosis. I am not sure this debate will ever be solved in the research, because so many factors come into play in your prognosis, as you can see from this chapter. However, people who maintain some sense of optimism appear to be more action oriented, and working closely with a medical team that truly supports your mental, physical, and spiritual health only further increases the probability of doing better. If your team helps in preventing and treating side effects as well as providing access to the standard or best of care, then it would seem this could improve prognosis. For example, reducing unnecessary delays in treatment can make a meaningful difference. Working with a good medical team is like being in a great marriage, family, or friendship, but working with an inadequate team or one not capable of addressing your beliefs, needs, or even not being open to your thoughts or other opinions is not a good recipe for short- or long-term success in your physical or mental health. Are you in a symbiotic healthy relationship or a chaotic unhealthy relationship? I believe most medical teams are symbiotic and healthy, but if chaotic, it may be time to look for other team members.

Still, again this is only half of the story because being a part of any good team suggests the relationship is bi-directional in terms of respect and expectations. In other words, as committed as your healthcare team should be toward you, it is important to ensure you are also doing everything realistically possible to enhance your own health via lifestyle changes, including dietary improvements, exercise, adequate rest or sleep, and mental health empowerment. This also helps create or sustain more of a positive attitude or mood to keep you going strong and fighting cancer to the best of your ability. You should rely and lean on a great team during your journey, but a great team should also expect great things and rely on you, too. This is the essence of a bi-directional medical team, which only further improves your probability of success.

34. You and Your Medical Team Part B. More Unique Opportunities and Access. Phase 1, 2, 3, and 4 Clinical Trials, Expanded/Early Access Programs (EAPs), Compassionate Use, Company Appeal Letters, Objective Off-Label Use or Non-Use, Insurance or Non-insurance assistance teams, etc.

A good relationship with your medical team also applies to when it may or may not be appropriate to get into a phase 1, 2, 3, or 4 clinical trial. These trials are occurring in AdvPCa every day locally, regionally, nationally, and globally. There are also Expanded/Early Access Programs (EAPs), and compassionate drug use programs offered by companies on a regular basis with a promising drug that appears to be on the path toward FDA or regulatory approval, that you may be able to access sooner or right now. There are also individual medical team compassionate use company appeal letters (emails) or requests, which allow some patients to receive an experimental drug when options are becoming more limited. The take home point here is your relationship with your medical team not only has an impact on your standard of care, or best options, but also your access to other novel opportunities. Thus, this relationship is believed to be the most important decision on your journey with AdvPCa. Again, most medical teams, in our opinion, are simply awe inspiring in terms of their dedication to patient care, but once in a while we also accept the fact there could be room for improvement or change.

PW Lifestyle Empowerment Moment

Another reason we believe your relationship with your medical team is so critical to your quality of life and prognosis is in two categories that need to receive more attention. The first involves "off-label and OTC or prescription medication utilization." Inquiries about potentially promising add-on, non-approved products to improve quality of life or prognosis is a gargantuan area of interest. Some of these have some preliminary (not definitive) merit. For example, the question of whether the cholesterol-lowering medication a person is using, or wanting to use, could help fight AdvPCa or improve prostate cancer prognosis when combined with standard of care treatments. How about a blood sugar or blood pressure drug? And then there are the countless dietary supplements where some rare medical teams dismiss these inquiries and never want the patient to deviate from the traditional course. On the opposite side, there are other teams who embrace these supplements almost too graciously.

In my opinion, the majority of medical teams are always open to the possibility of adding in other things, but with admirable objectivity, which is my hope for you. It is important to realize when trying to add something into the treatment mix that it could help, harm, or do nothing. If it is more likely to help and not harm you, and you require this product anyway for your overall or heart health, such as cholesterol lowering medication, then why not? If it could harm you, and it is not required for your overall health, then why? This was briefly touched on in prognosis indicator number nine, but more emphasis is needed here.

For example, not long ago the American Society of Clinical Oncology (ASCO), one of the most reputable oncology organizations in the world, produced a published clinical guideline statement suggesting a specific type of supplement (acetyl-L-carnitine or ALC) should not be used when trying to prevent the side effect known as "chemotherapy-induced peripheral neuropathy" (CIPN). The suggestion from past clinical studies was that this supplement could potentially increase the risk of this side effect when combined with certain types of chemotherapy (e.g., taxane drugs such as Taxotere—also known as "docetaxel"). So, why even try it when receiving chemotherapy? Separately, it has been more than a decade since some high-dose vitamin E supplements from the phase 3 SELECT prostate cancer prevention trial were found to increase the risk of this cancer, so why use it in high dosages now? In the meantime, there was a phase-3-like study organized primarily by Mayo Clinic researchers conducted on a supplement (Pure Ground Root of American-Wisconsin Ginseng certified and donated by the "Ginseng Board of Wisconsin" at a 3% ginsenoside concentration). The study, which enrolled patients from 40 medical institutions, potentially found that this supplement could reduce cancer-related fatigue (CRF) vs placebo, within 8 weeks, and had a low rate of side effects similar to the placebo used in the trial. So, why not discuss potentially using this one with your medical team if needed? Furthermore, the ongoing research suggests exercise has worked about as well as anything else out there to reduce CRF. How about the use of calcium and/or vitamin D supplements for bone health or to help prevent hypocalcemia when a patient is not able to achieve the recommended daily intakes from food and beverages? In other words, a great medical team should be open to discussing these off-label products with objectivity.

PW Lifestyle Empowerment Moment (another one even more unique)

Last, but not least, your medical team could also help you with other options, for example diverse resources or contacts, such as social workers and other patient advocates, who could assist you in looking for discounts or donations from some companies to help with your medical treatment or care. Most major drug or pharmaceutical companies also offer patient financial counselors with insurance assistance advice, or recommendations on how to reduce your financial burden or obligation (whether you have insurance or not), and these contact numbers are usually easy to locate on the official specific drug/company website. Who knew that you or your partner searching official medication websites for more information and assistance would be a lifestyle empowerment tip? But it is, and I encourage you to take advantage of this assistance!

35. Bonus or Miscellaneous Prognostic Factors ("Finding health where you and your medical team did not know it existed")

No book could give complete credibility to the countless prognosis indicators, and there are always new ones that are being appreciated (e.g., other new and older blood or tissue tests), or other less tangible ones that need to be recognized. All of this should be discussed with the medical team you entrust with your health. I also like to use the phrase "find health where you did not know it existed" to bring attention to all the parameters that do not appear on a medical chart or prognosis list. Everyone has their own thought, place, or action that could improve their physical, mental or spiritual health that is uniquely you. It could be a hobby, volunteering, mentorship at a support group meeting, walking more each day, less negative themed TV or internet, and more focus on strengthening or celebrating specific relationships. I think it's important for everyone reading this book to ask themselves where they can find health where they did not know it existed. It could involve getting out of your comfort zone and trying something different, which brings you to a healthier place such as attending a cooking, art, or dance class with your partner, or perhaps trying a new diet or exercise program. Whatever it is, and wherever it comes from, there will always be many prognostic parameters or educational tips that never get appreciated or recognized in a medical meeting or journal, but we all know they exist out there, and they are ready to be passionately embraced, or as I often say, "bear hugged." So, where do you or your medical team think you and your partner can find health where you or they did not know it existed? This is why the bonus open-ended tip was included below.

36. BONUS. Other tips or prognosis indicators wanting to discuss or already discussed with my medical team and overall support network include:

_____

_____

_____

_____

_____

_____

_____

Note: *The summary table of the 35+ potential prognosis indicators was important enough to place not only at the beginning of this chapter, but also at the end for easier or better access.*

_____
_____
_____
_____
_____
_____
_____
_____
_____
_____
_____
_____
_____
_____
_____
_____
_____
_____
_____
_____
_____
_____
_____
_____
_____
_____
_____
_____
_____
_____
_____
_____

35+ Promoting Wellness Tips or Potential Prognosis Indicators from A to Z that You Could Discuss with your Healthcare Team Before, During or After any Treatment

1. Age

2. Albumin blood test

3. Alkaline phosphatase (ALP) blood test

4. Asymptomatic or symptomatic cancer

5. Bone metastasis and/or number or volume of bone metastasis & oligometastatic prostate cancer (OMPC)

6. Bone-protecting agents (BPAs) & bone healthy behaviors

7. Circulating tumor cell (CTC) blood tests

8. Comorbidities and your medical history/other tests

9. Diet, exercise, sleep quality & quantity, stress reduction, and other lifestyle changes & even OTC medicine interests

10. Germline (your inherited cellular-genetic information since birth) and/or somatic (your cancer) biomarker testing—personalized or precision medicine

11. Gleason total score, Gleason grade group, or primary Gleason score from a pathology report

12. Health disparities, race, ethnicity, & your medical team

13. Hemoglobin/hematocrit/white blood cell/platelet counts-CBC (Complete Blood Count) test & the N:L ratio (bone marrow quality & quantity)

14. Hormone reduction treatment choice (ADT, LHRH, newer daily antagonist pills, or surgical testicular removal)

15. Imaging test results over time— pictures of the inside of the body (bone scan, MRI, PET/CT, etc.) & what and when you eat and exercise (lifestyle) could impact your results

16. Lactate/Lactic Acid Dehydrogenase (LDH) blood test

17. Mental health (stress, anxiety, depression, & associated conditions or issues)

18. Pain	29. Total testosterone (TT) levels before ADT
19. Partner/life partner/support network (it's a couple's disease)	30. Visceral (organs) and/or other soft-tissue disease spread (lymph nodes, organs, organ systems)
20. Performance status (ECOG, etc.)	
21. Preventive vaccines (vaccine preventable Illnesses) for adults including COVID-19	31. Volume (amount) of cancer & quantity/number of sites with cancer—Oligometastatic prostate cancer (OMPC) revisited
22. Previous responses to treatment(s) and/or how well you're able to tolerate treatment(s)	32. Weight loss (excessive/extreme) or the inability to gain weight when needed
23. Primary tumor site status & treatment, debulking, or "local control" of an advanced cancer	33. You and your medical team Part A. Bi-directional or symbiotic relationship—as important as it gets.
24. PSA & PSA kinetics (PSADT=PSA Doubling Time, PSAV=PSA Velocity, stable PSA, % PSA reductions, etc.)	34. You and your medical team Part B. Even more personalized unique opportunities, access, and assistance with your situation (clinical trials, EAPS, compassion use, appeal letters, insurance issues, etc.)
25. Sarcopenia severity (quality, quantity, & function)	
26. Spiritual health	35. Z = Miscellaneous. Finding health where you and your team did not know it existed.
27. Stage of cancer ("how far it has spread in the body")	
28. Time from initial treatment to AdvPCa diagnosis, or time on ADT before progressing (converting) to CRPC.	36. Bonus. Other Tips or Prognosis Indicators discussed with your medical team & overall support network include: _____

Bone-Protecting Agents (BPAs), Better Bone Health & Preventing and Treating Other ADT Side Effects from A-Z

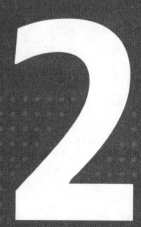

Promoting Wellness Quick & Concise Chapter Message

Xgeva (denosumab) and Zometa (zoledronic acid) are the two bone-protecting agents (BPAs) approved for use in some prostate cancer patients. A head-to-head phase 3 clinical trial of over 1900 patients from 342 medical centers in 39 countries was published many years ago and indicated that Xgeva appeared to work better compared to Zometa to protect bones and reduce skeletal-related events (SREs) or symptomatic skeletal events (SSEs). However, either drug works very well. If a doctor recommends these drugs before or after initiating ADT/AdvPCa treatment, then a patient would receive one or the other (usually Xgeva, but there are exceptions because again either drug works well). Xgeva is given as a subcutaneous (under the skin) injection and Zometa is given intravenously (IV) for no less than 15 minutes. Although neither drug has proven to improve overall survival in AdvPCa patients they can have a major impact on improving quality of life. Also, reducing SREs and SSEs prevents delays in treatment, which arguably could improve the prognosis of some patients.

Encouraging a normal daily intake of calcium and vitamin D was part of the primary recommendations in the Xgeva and Zometa clinical trials that ultimately resulted in the FDA approval of these drugs. When working with your medical team (including a dietician in some cases), if you cannot achieve adequate intakes from diet then supplemental calcium and/or vitamin D could be used to make up for the difference. The recommended daily intake of calcium and vitamin D is based on your age—generally 1000 mg of calcium and 600 IU (15 mcg) of vitamin D daily for adult men up to age 70, and 1200 mg calcium and 800 IU (20 mcg) of vitamin D daily for those 71 and older. In some cases, a vitamin D blood test (also known as "25-OH" vitamin D test) could be used to further determine your needs. Excessive intakes of calcium and vitamin D supplements can increase the risk of kidney stones and/or constipation, so please check with your medical team to make sure you need one or both of these supplements before taking them.

Bone loss is one potential side effect of ADT. This and other side effects should be discussed with your medical team, as well as what you can do to prevent or alleviate them.

Xgeva, Zometa and Bone Health

Bone is normally very active—slightly building up and breaking down throughout our lives. But aging, ADT and prostate cancer can have a major impact on bone quality and quantity, which makes it an important topic to discuss with your medical team.

Although it doesn't often appear so on a plain x-ray, bone is dynamic and constantly changing, ever so slightly breaking down and building up every second of the day. There are two types of cells that bone primarily relies on to build healthy new bone—osteoblasts and osteoclasts. The osteoblasts help to build new bone and act to simply "fill in tiny potholes on the road," so to speak. In contrast, the osteoclasts help create some of these small potholes to allow bones to further secure and strengthen more vulnerable areas. In other words, in healthy bones, osteoclasts function to break down bone so that osteoblasts can put healthier bone back in areas of the bone that need repair. This is the amazing yin and yang or bone balance that occurs throughout life to help keep your bones strong and healthy.

While Xgeva and Zometa block the ability of osteoclasts to function, they simply work in different ways. The goal of both is to stop the skeleton from losing more bone and, in the process, possibly build a little new healthy bone. This is much-needed good news because aging and ADT reduce bone quality and quantity, and prostate cancer has the unique ability to abnormally accelerate osteoclastic function, causing unhealthy amounts of bone imbalance, break down and loss. Furthermore, prostate cancer simultaneously increases the tendency of cancer-controlled and created osteoblasts to build abnormally weak bone. In fact, bone metastatic sites are often osteoblastic lesions. However, these bone metastatic sites are more chaotic and disorganized, and are not strong bone sites, which means they are more prone to subsequent problems. It is these areas of abnormal osteoblastic function that could be detected by imaging tests. It is for these reasons prostate cancer was and is still known as an "osteoblastic bone disease" when it invades the bones.

Why the bones? In theory, prostate cancer gravitates to bone because of a variety of compounds that not only potentially attract it, but help it function and survive better in bony areas. Researchers are constantly looking at ways to not just block the signals cancer uses to be attracted to bone, but also block other signals tumors use to survive and thrive on or within bone. Still, by reducing the ability of the osteoclasts to do an abnormal amount of damage, Xgeva and Zometa are effective at reducing bone loss from aging, ADT, or cancer, and by preventing and delaying skeletal related events (SREs) and symptomatic skeletal events (SSEs). Yet, what exactly are SREs or SSEs, and why are they such a large part of the reason these and other drugs are so important in some cases before or after CRPC occurs?

Skeletal-Related Event (SREs) or Symptomatic Skeletal Events (SSEs)—Many types exist with the goal of preventing all of them via better bone health.

Several problems can occur when cancer goes into the bones (not only bone fractures), so researchers decided to collectively refer to these as "skeletal-related events" (SREs). When these problems cause symptoms in a patient then some refer to them as "symptomatic skeletal events" (SSE) because they can potentially be more problematic in some cases. The different types of SREs or SSEs from past clinical studies (especially the first four) caused by metastatic prostate cancer include:

Bone fractures
These are known as "pathologic bone fractures" of the spine (vertebral area) or non-spine area (such as hip, leg, or wrist). In general, the most common sites for bone fractures are the hip, spine, wrist, and ribs. These are called pathologic fractures because they were not caused by an accident or trauma, but rather the tumor itself and/or the ADT treatment, which can

accelerate bone loss. Thus, it is important again to mention the impact of ADT, or minimal-to-no testosterone, which can reduce bone quantity and quality essentially making it easier for a bone to fracture, or for a tumor to cause further damage. This important point needs to be reiterated—protecting your bones when dealing with AdvPCa is extremely important because it protects a patient from a major side effect of ADT (bone loss), as well as the potentially damaging effects of the tumors themselves. So, there is a 2-for-1 benefit, or a 3-for-1 benefit in some cases because, as mentioned earlier, some men are also at higher risk of bone loss or fracture before they begin ADT because of their age and other issues that could be accelerating bone loss (e.g., other inflammatory diseases, chronic steroid medication use, physical inactivity, family history, etc.).

The need for radiation to the bone or an IV drug

When cancer penetrates the bone then it has the potential to cause pain. Therefore, some patients need radiation delivered to that same site to reduce the bone pain and potentially stop the tumor from doing more damage. This is known as "spot radiation." Other patients may require or get a benefit from a radiopharmaceutical drug (also known as a "radioisotope"), which are medications usually given intravenously (IV) that travel through the body, find those specific bone tumors, and then deliver a quick burst of damaging energy to them, which can also reduce or eliminate the pain from those sites. (Please see the chapter on Xofigo, a radiopharmaceutical, and information on the new radio-ligand therapy Lutetium-177/Pluvicto.)

Spinal cord compression

If prostate cancer gets into the backbone or spinal cord, it can create pressure and cause nerve damage. The nerves of the spinal cord control all kinds of bodily functions, so damage to the spinal cord could cause problems such as pain, numbness, muscle weakness, and even bladder control issues.

Surgery to the bone

If the bones become weak, damaged, or broken, they could require some type of specialized (orthopedic) surgery to repair the specific problematic bone site.

Hypercalcemia vs. Hypocalcemia

It is also important to mention a condition called "Hypercalcemia" (abnormally high blood level of calcium), which can occur with bone loss. Some researchers consider this an SRE because in certain instances it could be caused by cancer in the bones and could result in many problems. However, Xgeva and Zometa do a very good job of preventing this problem. In fact, these drugs are now used in some non-cancer-related emergency situations when a blood level of calcium becomes high enough to create a potentially life-threatening situation. In fact, one of the side effects of Xgeva or Zometa in cancer patients is actually "Hypocalcemia,"—the opposite problem, where the blood levels of calcium can get too low.

Need to change treatment because of an SRE

In some older studies of SREs or SSEs, they found it necessary to change cancer treatment to treat bone pain. In other words, many of these issues can be prevented with newer BPAs used today. Regardless of the criteria of what constitutes an SRE, it is now known these drugs prevent SREs, and in some cases SSEs.

> ### *PW Lifestyle Empowerment Moment*
>
> In the official prescribing information materials for the drug Xgeva it states the following: "Administer calcium and vitamin D as necessary to treat or prevent hypocalcemia." Again, another side effect, especially when starting these medications, is their ability to reduce your calcium blood levels, sometimes to an unhealthy low level (as mentioned previously). Therefore, part of the reason to normalize your dietary and supplemental intake of calcium and vitamin D is not only for proper bone health to support what the drug itself is doing (i.e., stopping bone loss), but also to help prevent low blood levels of calcium known as "hypocalcemia." At the same time, you do not want to get

an excessive amount of supplemental calcium or vitamin D because this could increase your risk of constipation and/or kidney stones. It is also interesting that in the prescribing information for Zometa it states the following: "Coadminister oral calcium supplements of 500 mg and a multiple vitamin containing 400 international units of vitamin D daily." In other words, the companies providing Xgeva and Zometa acknowledged the importance of normalizing your intake of calcium and vitamin D (first via diet and/or then supplements to make up the difference). While Xgeva appears to emphasize it more to prevent a side effect of their drug, Zometa seems to emphasize it more to help further reduce bone loss.

Remember the actual adult male recommendations for calcium are approximately (differs slightly based on the expert organization) 1000 mg/day total in adult males up to the age of 70 and 600 IU/day (15 mcg/day) of vitamin D, and for those 71 and older it is 1200 mg/day and 800 IU/day (20 mcg/day).

There has also been a debate concerning greater weight or higher body mass index (BMI) and bone drug effectiveness. Although these drugs appear to work just as well in overweight and obese individuals, it is interesting that regarding Xgeva, the steady state drug exposure was reported by the company to be greater in individuals of normal or moderate weight, versus heavier weight individuals. In addition, one well-known clinical study found slightly better increases in bone mineral density (BMD) at the hip, spine, and wrist in men with essentially a normal BMI versus those with higher BMIs. While this is interesting information, it probably results in minimal clinical differences or outcomes. Regardless, the take home message is there are numerous reasons to maintain a healthy weight/waist or prevent excessive weight gain for overall head-to-toe health, and this also appears to be the case for bone health.

Xgeva vs. Zometa

The Phase 3 Comparison Clinical Trial showed Xgeva was more effective in delaying or preventing skeletal-related events (SREs) or symptomatic skeletal events (SSEs), but the pros and cons of these drugs should still be discussed with your medical team.

A study called "20050103" (also known as "NCT00321620") of Xgeva vs. Zometa in men with metastatic CRPC found an overall reduction or delay in SREs (need for radiation to bone, pathological fracture, surgery to bone, or spinal cord compression) or SSEs (in general, symptoms occurring from these SREs) in favor of Xgeva over Zometa. Both drugs worked well in protecting bones, but Xgeva was more effective in preventing SREs and SSEs or delaying the time in experiencing an SRE or SSE versus Zometa. Additionally, it should be kept in mind that in general these drugs do not appear to impact PSA levels or overall survival.

Interestingly, the authors of this trial wrote, "We strongly recommended that all patients take daily supplemental calcium (>500 mg) and vitamin D (>400 IU)." There was significantly higher risk of hypocalcemia from Xgeva compared to Zometa in this study, which was essentially the only statistically significant difference between the two drugs in terms of safety. It tended to occur in the first six months of treatment and most of the cases were asymptomatic (without symptoms).

Osteonecrosis of the jaw (ONJ), a rare side effect of both drugs, occurred in 1-2% of the patients, but in slightly more patients on Xgeva. The problem with Zometa was that it did not work better than Xgeva, and it needs to be given intravenously and kidney function needs to be monitored because it could cause injury to this organ in some patients. In fact, before Zometa was used at its current dosage there was a much higher dosage (twice the amount) being tested in a previous study to see if it was more efficacious versus the current dosage, but it caused more kidney injuries, so it was not sold or used in prostate cancer. Also, there were more cases of "acute phase reactions" or temporary flu-like symptoms for a few days, especially after the first dosage with Zometa versus Xgeva. For these and other reasons, Xgeva is more likely to be used in prostate cancer versus Zometa when needed, but again this decision is up to you and your medical team. For instance, some patients do not tolerate Xgeva, so Zometa is used and vice versa. Some experts think the risk of hypocalcemia and the higher risk of ONJ should allow for select patients to receive Zometa.

Perhaps the most unappreciated reason to have a discussion with your healthcare team about using one of these drugs to protect your bone health is something else reflected in this phase 3 study, along with other major studies, which needs more attention. Some patients still dealt with some type of SRE while on these medications, despite such a significant reduction in risk for most patients. (Of course, there is a higher risk when doing nothing or taking a placebo.) In other words, these drugs work very well to protect patients from SREs, but SREs are still quite common. A pertinent analogy could be the following: car accidents and injuries ("SREs") are still common even if someone uses a seat belt ("bone-protective agent" or BPA), but at least there is a lower probability of being severely injured when wearing a seatbelt versus not wearing a seatbelt, which is why it is far better to wear a seat belt. The good news is these bone drugs also delayed the time to a first or subsequent SRE, so they not only prevent them from happening, but delay them until a later time in many patients, even if they were going to occur. The other piece of good news is the increased approval of more direct cancer treatment drugs for CRPC (see the rest of this book) not only results in the reduced progression of this disease, but also more reductions in SRE events. In other words, the combination of bone drugs and the better direct drug treatments for CRPC helps further reduce the risk and impact of these SREs.

Xgeva (also known as "denosumab")—Basics and Prolia

This drug is given as a subcutaneous (under the skin,) injection usually in the upper arm, upper thigh, or abdomen. It does an excellent job of stopping bone loss or injury during ADT or CRPC, but it must be given on a regular basis. For example, every four weeks, but this time period can vary based on what you and your medical team decide is best for you.

It works well in stopping bone loss because it is a human IgG2 monoclonal antibody that binds to and blocks a site in the human body known as "RANKL," which is a protein that normally helps osteoclasts break down bone and release calcium in the blood. Thus, by blocking this site it does not allow many osteoclasts to continue to break down bone. Osteoblasts are cells in the bone that help build bone, so if the osteoclasts are blocked from doing their job, then the osteoblasts are allowed to continue to work. This is why these drugs are so effective at not only stopping bone loss, but in some cases potentially increasing bone density at various sites in the body.

Xgeva helps prevent skeletal related events (SRE) in patients with bone metastasis from prostate cancer, and it is also approved for abnormally high levels of blood calcium levels that occur in some cancer patients ("hypercalcemia of malignancy") that does not respond to other treatments. Zometa is also approved for this situation.

This same drug (denosumab) is given to prevent bone loss in many women and in men with and without prostate cancer and is known as "Prolia." Prolia comes in a lower dosage (half as much) and is only needed two times a year. In fact, Prolia is also approved as a treatment to increase bone mass in men at high risk for fracture receiving ADT for nonmetastatic prostate cancer. Another advantage of Xgeva or Prolia is the ability to improve bone mineral density (BMD) not only at the spine and hip, but also at the wrist, which is one of the most common sites of fracture in the general population.

Zometa (also known as "zoledronic acid")— Basics and Reclast

Zometa is a drug in the "bisphosphonate" drug class, which is one of the largest groups of medications used to prevent bone loss. It is given as a single intravenous (IV) infusion over no less than 15 minutes. It also inhibits osteoclastic bone cells, so bones do not break down as easily, allowing osteoblasts to help build some new bone. Zometa ("zoledronic acid") was the primary bone-protective drug given to CRPC patients until Xgeva was approved. In fact, it is still used today in some osteoporotic men without prostate cancer to increase bone mass (and in some women), but it is a slightly higher dosage of zoledronic acid given just once a year. This drug is known as "Reclast." As mentioned earlier, it must be given by IV, and patients with a history of kidney problems may not be good candidates for this drug. There have been some reports of "bronchoconstricton" or breathing problems in aspirin-sensitive patients receiving zoledronic acid, so please tell your medical team if you are sensitive to aspirin.

On your IV treatment day you should be eating and drinking normally, and then drink at least two glasses of fluid, preferably water, within a few hours before the infusion. Ask your medical team if you can use acetaminophen (Tylenol) to reduce side effects of this treatment for a few days after you receive the infusion, as some patients experience flu-like symptoms.

The Catch—The uncommon or rare, but serious side effects of Xgeva or Zometa are ONJ and/or AFF

Both drugs have relatively similar safety or side effect profiles. However, two side effects, which are extremely rare but serious, need to be discussed. Though uncommon, these side effects garner a lot of attention, and are updated regularly in terms of prevention and treatment as more is discovered. The good news, again, is not only are they rare, but with greater awareness, including in this book, we hope the risk can be further reduced.

The two rare side effects of not only Xgeva or Zometa, but most bone protective drugs in these same respective drug classes are ONJ or AFF:

Osteonecrosis of the Jaw (also known as "ONJ")

The problem occurs when an upper or lower area of the teeth or jaw becomes infected, and this infection becomes difficult to cure while you are on these drugs. One way to reduce the risk of developing ONJ is to get dental clearance or a clean bill of health from a dentist and/or your oral surgeon before starting Xgeva or Zometa. Ask your medical/dental team to perform an oral examination before starting Xgeva or Zometa and conduct periodic exams while you are on these or any bone drugs. If you should need invasive dental work while on these drugs, then ask your medical/dental team if a bone "drug holiday" is needed— some time away from these bone medications until after the dental procedure heals.

That bears repeating: No invasive dental procedures (e.g., tooth extraction, dental implants, oral surgery, etc.) should be attempted while on this drug without a discussion with your dental/medical team. Also ask your physician if your bone imaging test indicates that you might be at a higher risk for ONJ. Most cases of ONJ occur in patients who have been treated for longer durations with these drugs, and commonly ONJ patients reported a previous invasive dental procedure such as tooth removal or insertion, use of a dental appliance, or even poor general oral hygiene. If you develop any of the following symptoms, be sure to check with your medical team right away:

- Chronic sinusitis (inflammation of the sinuses)
- Foul-smelling drainage in the jaw area
- Mouth or facial pain that resembles a toothache
- Numbness in either the upper or lower jaw area
- Persistent discomfort or pain and/or slow healing of the mouth or jaw after a dental procedure or surgery
- An exposed bony area inside the mouth when looking in the mirror

Again, although it has received a good deal of media attention, this is a rare side effect. Most phase 3 clinical trials reported a rate of 1-2% risk during the studies. However, with more awareness and early detection patients can lower this risk even further. Please consult your medical team regarding your personal risk and prevention advice.

> ### PW Lifestyle Empowerment Moment
>
> Better oral hygiene, including fixing poor-fitting dentures or any other dental appliance, could reduce the risk of ONJ even further. In addition, unhealthy habits such smoking, tobacco use, or excessive alcohol intake can increase the risk of ONJ, as well as other health issues. Heart healthy = Dental Healthy! The ability to prevent ONJ by taking care of yourself and your teeth cannot be overestimated. Again, the use of any dental appliances including bridges, braces/retainers, crowns, dentures, fillings, mouth guards, prosthetics, and airway opening devices to reduce snoring or obstructive sleep apnea (OSA) could potentially increase the risk of ONJ.

Atypical Femur Fractures (AFF)

Atypical femur fractures, which are also known as "atypical subtrochanteric and diaphyseal femoral fractures" or "unusual thigh bone fractures," are stress type fractures occurring rarely in the upper part of the femur ("thighbone") which is the longest and strongest bone in the body. These fractures occur with no or minimal stress or trauma to that area, for example, a fall from a standing height or less. They can occur in individuals whether they are taking these bone medications or not. The reason AFF even occurs is not well understood, but it may be related to a build-up of bone micro-damage in some individuals, which does not get adequately repaired by the body and results in these specific stress fractures. Anatomical or geometrical differences in human femurs and even genetic predisposition may also play a role.

There are numerous risk factors for AFF being studied now including a higher risk in women, individuals of Asian descent, those using multiple bone drugs at once, patients using zoledronic acid then using denosumab later (probably vice versa also), use of stronger steroid medications ("glucocorticoids"), inflammatory co-morbidities (e.g., rheumatoid arthritis), diabetes. low blood levels of calcium or vitamin D, younger age, increased BMI, and rare genetic diseases. All these factors could be associated with a higher risk of AFF. In general, the longer and more often a person needs these drugs, the greater the risk of AFF (similar to ONJ). However, to place the risk in perspective, it is estimated that for every 100 fractures prevented there is approximately one AFF that occurs. Another review found 50-130 cases per 100,000 people with use of these drugs for more than five years. Other recent clinical reviews also suggest a 1-2% risk, with more than 3.5 to 4 years, or more than 1.5 to 8 years of bone medication use raising the risk of AFF. Basically, some experts are calling for an assessment of risk every two years. Yet, many of these statistics are for non-cancer patients receiving these drugs.

Interestingly, for patients receiving these drugs for bone metastases, the incidence of AFF has reported to be lower, at 0.05 cases per 100,000 people or approximately 0.5% incidence. This may be due to the concentration of these drugs at metastatic sites, which allows other areas to heal adequately (a theory). It may also be lower because there was less awareness or recognition of the problem in cancer patients, which is changing quickly. Therefore, please ask your medical team about the latest risk statistics, because until recently most of what was known about these risks were primarily from studies of women on these medications. Also, please keep in mind that any unusual dull or aching thigh, hip, or groin pain should be discussed with your medical team. Ask your team if you need an imaging study or picture of the femur area if you are at high-risk for AFF or experiencing these symptoms.

Newer research also suggests that ONJ and AFF are not necessarily independent or separate entities in some cases and could be part of an even more rare potential cluster of problems that might occur with Xgeva, Zometa or similar oral, injectable, and IV drugs in their class (Fosamax/alendronate, Prolia, Reclast, etc.). If you are at high risk for either ONJ or AFF, or diagnosed with either condition, then please ask your medical team if you should be assessed or evaluated for the risk of the other condition. In other words, if you are at risk for ONJ or diagnosed with ONJ please ask your team if you should be evaluated for AFF and vice versa.

PW Lifestyle Empowerment Moment

Most updated clinical reviews suggest paying close attention to normalizing calcium and vitamin D intake for AFF prevention. There should also be attention given to any other medications contributing to an increased risk of bone loss to determine if some can be reduced, or even modified. If an AFF occurs, then the other femur without AFF should also be evaluated because in about one quarter to one third of AFF cases the other femur showed signs of risk for AFF.

More Common Side Effects of Xgeva or Zometa—

and prescription pills (alendronate = Fosamax, ibandronate = Boniva, risedronate = Actonel, etc.) are an option in rare cases.

Most of the side effects of these drugs are mild, or temporary, and if any continue or increase in severity talk to your healthcare team. For example, common side effects of a short-duration include fever or flu-like reaction such as chills, weakness, and muscle, bone, and joint aches soon after treatment. Back, muscle, and joint pain were more common in men with prostate cancer treated with these medications. Other side effects include gastrointestinal problems (e.g., constipation), anemia, nausea, fatigue, and loss of appetite. If you have a kidney problem or an irregular heartbeat, Xgeva or Zometa can make it worse in some rare cases. It should also be noted that if for any reason a person cannot receive the injection or IV forms of BPAs then there is a long list of potential prescription pill options (alendronate = Fosamax, ibandronate = Boniva, risedronate = Actonel, etc.).

Although these drugs were not tested as rigorously in prostate cancer, and especially CRPC, compared to the injection or IV BPAs, it would still be better to use a BPA in many of these cases than none at all. In other words, the prescription pill options at least have a preliminary track record of slowing or stopping bone loss while on ADT.

PW Bone Health Summary and Checklist

There is even more information on bone health in the diet and supplements chapter. However, since this chapter promotes bone health, we included a checklist of items here to think about and discuss with your medical team. Remember, receiving a drug for bone health can occur before or during ADT, or when dealing with CRPC, but there are many other bone health items that ideally should receive attention, including:

- **DEXA (dual-energy x-ray absorptiometry)**—This is a special type of open (not enclosed) low radiation exposure machine used throughout the world for men and women as a part of a larger checklist to determine if their bones are healthy. Keep in mind this is completely different from a bone scan used in some cases to find metastatic bone sites. The DEXA scan only takes 10-20 minutes and is not confining or claustrophobic like an MRI, but open. The device looks generally at your spine, hip and more rarely the wrist. DEXA scans also have the ability, in some cases, to measure body fat and are used in many studies of lifestyle changes, including diet or pills and their impact on weight loss. DEXA scans generate what is known as a T-score and based on this score you can be diagnosed with normal, osteopenia, or osteoporotic bones or osteoporosis when compared to someone of a younger age and gender. You will also receive a Z-score, which ideally compares you to someone of your own age and gender. Once the DEXA, or another imaging device for bone mineral density (BMD) measurement is completed then your medical team can tell you more about your bone health. In fact, once your hip, or in reality your

"Femoral Neck BMD" is measured by an imaging device it can be used in one of the most commonly accessed Internet bone health questionnaires in the world known as the Fracture Risk Assessment Tool or FRAX (**sheffield.ac.uk/FRAX/index.aspx**).

- **FRAX** is a 12-question assessment tool that takes 30 seconds to approximately one minute to answer, which can help provide your future probability or risk of a major osteoporosis-related fracture or a hip fracture. FRAX also incorporates past data from where you live globally and your race, before moving to the official questionnaire. But remember these are just general guidelines and may, in fact, underestimate your risk. The first 11 questions of FRAX asks for your:

  - Age
  - Sex
  - Weight
  - Height
  - Previous fracture history
  - If a parent fractured a hip
  - Whether or not you smoke
  - Use of steroid medications
  - Having been diagnosed with rheumatoid arthritis or not
  - If you have another (secondary) form of osteoporosis (for example, from ADT)
  - Alcohol intake

Question 12 then asks you to enter your femoral neck BMD (in g/cm2) usually from the imaging device company on your BMD DEXA report (e.g., GE, Hologic, Norland, etc.). FRAX helps many medical teams decide whether to recommend an osteoporosis drug, and theoretically it can play a role in prostate cancer bone medication treatment for some men receiving ADT.

PW Lifestyle Empowerment Moment

Perhaps one the greatest unappreciated FRAX questionnaire contributions is that it emphasizes that bone health is about more than just taking a drug. Many factors come into play to promote better bone health. Factors such as family history, medications (e.g., some steroid drugs may increase risk), alcohol use (higher intake = higher risk), tobacco use (increases risk), and other inflammatory conditions can all impact bone health and should be considered when discussing risk of bone problems with your medical team. We have included these factors and more in your bone health checklist. For example, resistance exercise is a well-known and researched method to improve or maintain BMD, but there is some controversy over whether patients with metastatic bone sites should lift weights because, as mentioned earlier in the chapter, these sites are associated with more vulnerable or weaker bone areas, which theoretically could be injured or even fracture when too much pressure is applied. This theory has not been well studied, but of course the concern makes sense. Still, there is some research to support some type of middle ground or light resistance activity, such as resistance bands or "yoga lite" could be beneficial in some cases. But, again, this decision should be individualized and discussed with your medical team. The rest of the bone health checklist is more self-explanatory.

PW Quick Bone Health Checklist
What to Ask Your Medical Team When It Comes to Bone Health

- Do I need any type of imaging test now or in the future, for example a DEXA, to determine if I have bone loss, osteopenia or osteoporosis in my hip and/or spine? Should you also look at other sites of potential bone loss such as my wrists?

- Do I need a drug now, or in the near future to protect my bones? (For example, Xgeva or another prescription medication.) And what is the latest prevention advice for the rare (ONJ, AFF) and more common side effects from these medications?

- Can I do some type of resistance exercise (e.g., weightlifting, resistance bands, yoga, etc.) to protect my bones, or is it too risky for my situation because of metastatic bone sites?

- Is there a dietician, another expert or website (see end of this chapter please for some suggested internet sites) you recommend, to evaluate my daily calcium and vitamin D intakes from diet and whether I need a supplement? If needed, what specific type of supplements and dosage is recommended? The generally accepted adult male recommendations for calcium and vitamin D are 1000 mg/day and 600 IU (15 mcg)/day up to the age of 70, and for those 71 years and older it is 1200 mg/day & 800 IU (20 mcg)/day. This is the total recommended daily amount or intake. (Ideally, these amounts should come from diet or diet and supplementation, if diet alone cannot achieve this goal.)

- Do I need a vitamin D (also known as 25-OH vitamin D) or other blood test (ALP, etc.) that could give some indication of my bone health?

- Do I need to do a Fracture Risk Assessment (FRAX) online evaluation of my bone health?

- Am I taking any other prescription medications or supplements that could be impacting my bone health for better or worse; and if for the worse, could they be modified or adjusted?

- Do I need to modify my home to prevent falls (e.g., move furniture away from walking areas, repair loose carpets or remove rugs, move any objects you could trip over)? Other fall prevention tips include making sure rooms are well lit, installing handrails in and around the bathtub or shower, and using non-slip mats in these areas.

What can I do right now to improve my own bone health?

- Reduce alcohol intake to moderate levels or eliminate

- Quit smoking or using tobacco products

- Adhere to a heart healthy diet because many other nutrients from these diets could be associated with better overall health, including bone health, such as: increasing dietary potassium, lowering sodium intake (if excessive), increasing dietary fiber, and making sure you are consuming adequate healthy dietary protein (beans, lentils, nuts, seeds, etc.) to support muscles, which support the bones.

- Try and get some type of aerobic or balance (Pilates, Tai Chi, Yoga, etc.) exercise daily, and add in some type of upper- and lower-body resistance exercises 2-3 times a week, if your medical team agrees that it is safe.

- Keep all other medical conditions (e.g., diabetes, heart disease, high blood pressure, etc.) under control, because they could increase the risk of bone loss based on the latest research. In some cases, normalizing heart healthy numbers, such as blood cholesterol levels, may also reduce bone loss.

- **Remember:** HEART HEALTHY = BONE HEALTHY!

> ### PW Lifestyle Empowerment Moment Bonus
>
> Additional resources for excellent bone healthy lifestyle tips, including how to accurately calculate or estimate your daily calcium intake, include the following:

- International Osteoporosis Foundation (**osteoporosis.foundation**)

- Bone Health & Osteoporosis Foundation (BHOF) (**bonehealthandosteoporosis.org**)

ADT Potential Side Effects from A-to-Z
PW Rapid Review & Reference (RRR)

(**Note:** *Also See Heart Healthy Awareness Material & More Empowerment Tips in the Appendix Section Under the 5Bs. Always talk to your medical team if you or your partner notice any new, worsening, or even improving side effects from ADT.*)

ADT Potential Side Effects From A-to-Z (Heart Healthy Lifestyle Changes = Less Potential ADT Side Effects)	Preventive and Treatment Options from Lifestyle, Supplements, Rx, and Other Interventions
Anemia	Mostly normocytic (normal size), normochromic (normal color) anemia, and often mild to moderate in severity and in general does not require medical intervention or supplementation. When testosterone levels are partially or fully restored then anemia values often improve. Most patients (approximately 90%) should expect some reduction in any of the following lab values: hematocrit, hemoglobin, and/or red blood cell count within the first 3-6 months of ADT treatment. For example, median hemoglobin decreases in some prospective studies was 1.2 g/dL. Regardless, checking for other causes of anemia can be done by your team if needed, but again this anemia is expected with ADT. No lifestyle changes or supplements can improve it unless the anemia is caused by something else (for example B12/folate or iron deficiency, which is rare). Separately, chemotherapy can also cause a reduction in blood counts (including red and white blood cells, platelets, etc.) and your healthcare team are experts in treating these and other ADT side effects.

Bone Loss (Osteopenia, osteoporosis) (PLEASE ALSO REFER TO THE BONE HEALTH EDUCATIONAL MATERIAL IN CHAPTER 2 OF THIS BOOK BEFORE THIS SPECIFIC TABLE)	• Aerobic exercise most days of the week and resistance exercise 2-3 times a week • Calculate daily dietary calcium and vitamin D intake to decide if any changes in dosages from diet ideally or supplements are needed. • Prescription medication should be addressed based on baseline bone health, ADT duration, DEXA scan, etc. Anyone starting or on ADT should have a conversation about when to get a DEXA scan (imaging test to help detect bone loss).
Cardiovascular disease (CVD) and type 2 diabetes, or increased cholesterol and/or pre-diabetes (blood sugar) and an association with metabolic syndrome (high triglycerides, low HDL, increased blood pressure, blood sugar, and waist circumference). [PLEASE SEE THE APPENDIX OF THIS BOOK FOR ADDITIONAL INFORMATION ON THIS SUBJECT]	• Lifestyle changes change lives (think heart healthy behaviors). • Statins and/or ezetimibe or PCSK9 inhibitors to lower cholesterol • Abnormal glucose levels could be controlled or reduced via lifestyle changes, but in some cases metformin or another prescription medication could be discussed. • Prescription fish oil (omega-3) to lower elevated triglycerides is FDA approved, but it is also currently somewhat controversial in terms of true clinical effectiveness over placebo in terms of reducing actual cardiovascular events in some patients. • Metabolic syndrome could be increased in patients on ADT and heart healthy behaviors and treatments can address these issues.
Cognitive Health or Cognitive Deficits and Dementia risk (PLEASE SEE THE BONUS COGNITIVE HEALTH TIPS THAT OCCUR RIGHT AFTER THIS TABLE IN THIS CHAPTER)	Controversial and recent research suggests some specific forms of ADT could increase the risk of some cognitive issues.

Fatigue (Also known as **"cancer-related fatigue"** or "CRF")	• It's important to repeat here that exercise continues to have some of the most consistent beneficial research in preventing and reducing CRF. • Aerobic and resistance exercise appears to work better than any drug thus far in clinical studies. Cognitive behavioral therapy (CBT) also works well. • Adequate recovery time from exercise • Moderate caffeine from beverages
Gynecomastia (Breast enlargement and/or pain or increased sensitivity)	• ADT can increase the risk of this situation, and although rarely problematic it can be prevented and treated in some cases with an anti-estrogen pill such as tamoxifen, or an "aromatase inhibitor," which blocks the ability of estrogen to stimulate the breast tissue. • The other effective preventive method is to receive a small dose of radiation to each breast (known as "prophylactic breast radiation"), and it takes minimal amounts of time and usually needs to be done one time. • Men who have already experienced significant breast enlargement also have the option of using a specialist (such as a plastic surgeon) to remove the excess tissue.
Hair Changes and/or Dry Skin	• Hair growth or slowing of hair loss on the scalp (yes, that's right), some hair loss on the rest of the body (arms, chest, neck, legs), and skin that feels more rough or dry from ADT. • Testosterone is often needed to continue to lose hair on the scalp as men age, but hair increases or continues to grow on other parts of the body. However, without testosterone, less loss of hair on the scalp and increased potential loss on the body could occur. This is not treated, but some forms of chemotherapy can cause hair loss on the scalp (including Taxotere or docetaxel).

Hair Changes and/or Dry Skin (continued)	• Dry air, cold air, indoor heating, friction, and even heavy clothing can make your skin dry, itchy, red, and susceptible to cracking. Long hot showers and baths are not a good idea unless you are with your significant other. Hot water removes the natural oils that the skin produces. Use a mild, moisturizing, and scent-free cleanser. Use warm rather than hot water. Keep the bathroom door closed to keep in the humidity, and do not dry your skin aggressively with a towel because your skin needs to be a little moist/wet when applying moisturizer. Wear soft clothes such as cotton and try to avoid rougher fabrics against your skin.
Hot Flashes (HF)/ Hot Flushes (HF) and/or Insomnia (Also known as "vasomotor symptoms", which includes "night sweats", which could be a cause of less sleep-insomnia. Thus, improving sleep could reduce the impact of HF, or even result in less medical treatment for hot flashes.) [PLEASE SEE THE BONUS HOT FLASH SECTION AFTER THIS TABLE IN THIS CHAPTER FOR MORE LIFESTYLE TIPS & YOUR OWN HOT FLASH DIARY. PLEASE ALSO SEE THE HEALTHY SLEEP RECOMMENDATIONS (appendix 5BB) IN THE APPENDIX OF THIS BOOK.]	• Maintaining a healthy weight could reduce the intensity or severity of HF. A healthy diet and exercise could also improve symptoms, including high intensity interval training (HIIT), if your medical team approves. • Flaxseed powder (2-3 tablespoons per day) has some initial efficacy data. • Acupuncture has good preliminary results. • No dietary supplement has found a consistent benefit over placebo. • Many prescription medicines (estrogen, progesterone, SNRI, SSRI, etc.) have side effect issues today, so talk to your healthcare team about the best and safest drug for you if needed. • Often, insomnia could also be an issue associated with ADT or caused by ADT, and this should be addressed by your healthcare team.

Mood Changes, disorders, and emotional responses (Emotional lability, stress, anxiety, depression, etc.) [PLEASE SEE THE APPENDIX OF THIS BOOK FOR ADDITIONAL INFORMATION ON THIS TOPIC]	• Studies continue to suggest the loss of testosterone could be associated with a variety of mood changes such as emotional lability, or abrupt changes in mood including increased sensitivity or even irritability. ADT could also be associated with increased stress, anxiety, or depression either by serving as a reminder of being treated for cancer, or in some patients could be caused by having low or no testosterone. • Exercise continues to provide diverse mental health benefits in ADT as well as other prostate cancer patients. • Talk to your healthcare team if you or your partner notice any mood or mental health changes.
Sarcopenia (Loss of muscle mass or size, strength and/or function) [PLEASE SEE THE BONUS RESISTANCE EXERCISE SECTION AFTER THIS TABLE IN THIS CHAPTER FOR MORE EXERCISE TIPS]	• Resistance exercise 2-3 times per week is the gold standard for prevention and treatment that no pill has matched or surpassed. • Preliminary evidence suggests protein powders/supplements could also assist muscle protein synthesis (MPS), but the current impact on ADT patients is unknown or of minimal benefit from preliminary studies. Creatine is also being tested in a clinical trial of patients on ADT so ask your healthcare team about the latest results.
Sexual Dysfunction (Erectile Dysfunction-ED, and/or loss of libido-sex drive) AND ask your medical team about **Penile Rehabilitation** for ED and the other related issues such as penis/scrotum (genital) shrinkage from ADT and other cancer therapies, which are also potentially improved by many of these same ED treatments.	• Most prostate cancer treatments have an ability to cause some degree of ED and/or libido problems. • Heart Healthy = Erection/libido healthy. Exercise, diet, improving your heart healthy behaviors and numbers could improve your sexual health. • Some supplements such as L-citrulline have been tested with some conventional treatments.

Sexual Dysfunction (continued)	• Prescription medications (PDE-5 inhibitor class such as Cialis, Levitra, Stendra, Viagra, etc.), vacuum erection devices (VED), intra-urethral suppository such as Muse (alprostadil), and/or penile injections of one or multiple medications have all been effective in many patients for penile rehabilitation and in treating ED. • Low-intensity shock wave therapy (LiSWT) is a new option being tested, but if your team thinks you should try it then please check prices first because it can be costly in some cases. • Penile prosthesis has been highly effective for some men not responding or not satisfied with other medical treatments, but like any of the other options, the pros and cons need to be reviewed with your healthcare team. • Penis/scrotum shrinkage can occur with several prostate cancer treatments from either ADT due to the reduction in testosterone, or nerve bundle injury near the prostate from other treatments. Reductions in the length and width of the penis can occur and/or a decrease in scrotum size. However, ED treatments listed earlier can stimulate and improve blood flow to these tissues and minimize or prevent these size changes, which is part of the reason "penile rehabilitation" refers to beneficially impacting a variety of sexual health areas and should be discussed with your healthcare team before, during, and after ADT or other prostate cancer treatments.
Weight/Waist Gain (Subcutaneous adipose tissue-right under the skin, and especially visceral adipose tissue increases including a potential increased risk of fatty liver) [PLEASE SEE THE APPENDIX OF THIS BOOK FOR ADDITIONAL INFORMATION ON THIS TOPIC]	• Lifestyle changes such as heart healthy diet, aerobic and resistance exercise • Metformin with dietary changes has some positive preliminary data with ADT for weight loss. Ask your medical team about the latest research on the class of medications known as glucagon-like peptide 1 (GLP-1) agonists, for example "semaglutide". They have resulted in significant weight loss for some patients not on ADT, but results in patients on ADT are expected soon.

Note: *Most side effects in this chapter can be prevented to some degree or improved with exercise along with medical treatment when needed. In addition, most of these side effects improve or resolve if testosterone recovers or increases back to a healthy level after ADT is discontinued. If you need to be on ADT continuously (for years) then it's imperative that you and your medical team review the latest options to prevent and treat these potential side effects. Please keep in mind that ADT is also used in patients with INTERMEDIATE and HIGH-RISK prostate cancer along with radiation therapy in those with earlier stages of CSPC (aka hormone sensitive prostate cancer). The average time ADT is given in intermediate disease in 4-6 months and the average time ADT is given in high-risk prostate cancer is 2-3 years. Although, the majority of ADT utilized in prostate cancer is for advanced prostate cancer. Therefore, ADT in this table not only refers to testosterone lowering medication, but also to the newer testosterone impacting medications known as the androgen receptor inhibitors (ARIs) and androgen synthesis inhibitors (ASIs) pills discussed in Chapter 4, which are now used in some cases for men with advanced prostate cancer whether they have advanced CSPC or CRPC.*

Cognitive Health Tips from A-to-Z
PW Rapid Review & Reference (RRR)

This table lists some of the most common lifestyle changes and health barometers associated with brain or cognitive health. Perhaps the best general advice to keep your brain healthy is to do whatever is practically possible to reduce your cardiovascular risk to as close to zero as possible (Heart Healthy = Mind/Brain Healthy).

Cognitive/Brain Health Risk factors From A-to-Z	Recommendation for Optimal Cognitive/Brain Health
Alcohol	Limit or eliminate it because alcohol use disorders are now the number one cause of preventable dementia!
BMI— weight/waist circumference	Healthy as possible to prevent unhealthy weight/waist gain (obesity)
Blood Cholesterol	Healthy as possible to prevent high cholesterol (dyslipidemia)
Blood Pressure	Healthy as possible to prevent hypertension
Blood Sugar	Healthy as possible to prevent diabetes or uncontrolled diabetes
Depression	Needs to be addressed and/or treated because when it's unaddressed and often untreated it can lead to cognitive problems.

Diet Quality	Increasing dietary quality from DASH, Mediterranean and even the MIND or other diets suggests improving diet quality is important in maintaining or improving cognitive health.
Exercise (Physical Activity)	Feeds an area of the brain known as the "hippocampus" to keep memory sharp. Regular exercise is now recommended in some clinical guidelines to potentially prevent dementia.
Family Health/ Disease Tree	Discuss your family history or genetic history with your healthcare team to see if you are at an increased risk of cognitive problems. An ApoE4 variant test is now conducted in some clinical settings to determine if there is an increased risk of Alzheimer's disease (AD).
Hearing Loss	Needs to be treated because if untreated it could lead to cognitive problems. Hearing aids when needed could preserve or improve memory.
Learning	Never ending brain stimulation through reading, crosswords, puzzles, card games, dancing, etc. because the brain needs to be stimulated to stay healthy ("use it or lose it").
Medications	Some medications such as anti-cholinergic drugs are associated with reduced cognitive health. Review your medications with your healthcare team for the latest update on which ones are more concerning. Also, google or search American Geriatric Society (AGS) "Beers Criteria" for an updated list of medications that could cause cognitive or other health issues with aging.
Sleep	Insomnia and sleep apnea are brain unhealthy. Better sleep clears the brain of metabolic waste products via the "glymphatic system."

Socialization	Isolation and loneliness have been associated with cognitive problems.
Tobacco	Tobacco may have a harmful effect on cognitive function, and it's just not heart healthy. Please eliminate.
Thyroid Hormone	Too low or too high levels (outside of the normal range) of thyroid hormone can be associated with memory issues.
Vitamin B12 blood test	Low blood levels of vitamin B12 is associated with memory issues. There are other vitamin (nutrients such as B1-thiamine) tests or medical conditions that can also be tested, which could also impact memory. However, those are often the result of other issues (e.g., alcohol), so that should be discussed with your healthcare team.

Note: *Whether ADT or another form of it (androgen receptor inhibitors-ARIs, androgen synthesis inhibitors-ASIs, etc.) increases the risk of cognitive issues is being researched, but ADT has been associated with some cognitive issues and regardless of the risk it should be something that at least receives more awareness and prevention tips. Also, see the Appendix for the 5Bs for more comprehensive information on being heart and mind healthy! Heart health = cognitive health!*

Hot Flash Lifestyle Reduction Tips from A-to-Z
PW Rapid Review & Reference (RRR)

Researchers have learned from studies of women going through menopause that lifestyle changes may play a large role in the management of hot flashes. Before deciding with your doctor about the proper treatment for your hot flashes, you need to determine the frequency and severity of the hot flashes.

Using the rating scale that follows, you can assess the situation with your hot flashes. Just use the journal pages that follow to record your hot flash history for discussion with your physician at your next visit. You may notice certain foods or activities that intensify the hot flashes and be able to make lifestyle changes that alleviate some of the occurrences.

Intensity/ Severity	Score	Length/ Duration	Observations
MILD **Hot Flash**	1 point	Less than 1 minute.	Warm & slightly uncomfortable, no perspiration.
MODERATE **Hot Flash**	2 points	Less than 5 minutes.	Warmth involving more of the body, perspiration, taking off some layers of clothing.
SEVERE **Hot Flash**	3 points	Greater than 5 minutes.	Burning warmth, disruption of normal life activities such as sleep or work, excessive perspiration, frequent thermostat changes in your house.
VERY SEVERE **Hot Flash**	4 points	Time is not an issue.	Complete disruption of normal activities to the point where it would make you consider discontinuing the androgen-deprivation treatment.

Personal Hot Flash Diary - Week 1

Date: _____

Weekday	# of daily hot flashes	Intensity/ Severity	Note on occurrences
Sunday			
Monday			
Tuesday			
Wednesday			
Thursday			
Friday			
Saturday			

Personal Hot Flash Diary - Week 2

Date: _____

Weekday	# of daily hot flashes	Intensity/ Severity	Note on occurrences
Sunday			
Monday			
Tuesday			
Wednesday			
Thursday			
Friday			
Saturday			

Lifestyle Changes: By using the hot flash diary and some of the following low-cost lifestyle options, you may expect to see a 25 to 50 percent reduction overall in those annoying hot flashes. These methods are not sufficient for severe hot flashes, which should be discussed with your healthcare team.

Lifestyle Change	Advantages & Disadvantages
Avoid hot beverages, spicy foods, and excess alcohol or caffeine.	Many foods and beverages can trigger hot flashes or make them worse. Your diary may help identify offenders for you.
Avoid smoking or breathing secondhand smoke.	Not only heart unhealthy, tobacco smoke makes hot flashes worse due to circulatory and temperature changes it produces in your body.
Controlled, deep, slow abdominal breathing (6–8 breaths per minute) for at least 15 minutes twice daily (morning, midday and/ or evening) or at the beginning of a hot flash.	Also known as "paced respiration," it has been shown to decrease blood pressure (temporarily), hot flashes, and the severity of a hot flash. However, this technique needs practice or it may need to be taught to you because it involves moving stomach muscles in and out.
Diet quality	Improving the quality of your diet by including more plant-based foods and reducing unhealthy processed foods is not only heart healthy but research suggests it may reduce hot flashes.
Keeping a diary.	Diary—keeping for just 2 to 4 weeks can give you the best insight into what does and does not impact your hot flashes. Give it a try!
Low-impact daily exercise.	Exercise has been shown to reduce stress, improve mood, and it may reduce hot flashes. Use a fan or work out in a cool location.
Stress reduction (meditation, relaxation techniques, yoga, etc.).	Relaxation exercises can help with flashes and may also improve other areas of your life, such as sleep.

Use cooling methods—ice-cubes, cool beverages, fan reducing room temperature, opening a window, chilling pillows and/or pillow coverings.	If your body's core temperature increases slightly it can trigger a hot flash so it just makes sense to keep yourself a bit cooler.
Wear loose-fitting clothing and layer clothing.	Helps to keep your body's core temperature slightly lower, and prevents clothing from feeling constricting when a hot flash occurs. Layers allow you to easily shed clothing to regulate temperature shifts.

Complementary and Alternative Treatments

It may be best to begin these prior to testosterone suppression, but you should check with your doctor before starting any treatment to be sure that they do not interfere with your cancer therapy. You would not want to consider more than one or two of these options at one time. As with the lifestyle changes, you might expect to see a 25 to 50 percent improvement using these treatments.

Complementary & Alternative Treatments	Advantages & Disadvantages
Acupuncture (1 to 2 times every week or two).	Minimal side effects from preliminary studies thus far, traditional needle and other forms of acupuncture have helped, not inexpensive.
Flaxseed Powder (2 to 3 tablespoons a day on foods or in beverages).	Cheap, high in fiber and omega-3 fatty acids, heart healthy, but lacks studies in men.
Soy Products/Protein (several servings a day or 20 to 40 grams of soy protein per day).	Cheap. Natural products (beans, powder, tofu) are heart healthy and may be more effective and healthy as compared to soy pills. As dosage is increased, so do gastrointestinal side effects.

Resistance Exercise Tips from A-to-Z
PW Rapid Review & Reference (RRR)

The following table includes some of the more common resistance exercises used in prostate cancer studies to help prevent muscle mass loss (sarcopenia) and bone loss. Only a few of each type of the resistance exercises below are needed two to three times each week. For example, some studies just used six types of total exercises per session such as: Chest press, latissimus pull-down, leg curl, leg extension, leg press, and seated row. These covered the upper and lower body adequately and patients still benefited from these shorter routines!

Upper Body Weightlifting/Resistance Exercises (from past studies)
Biceps Curl
Chest Press
Latissimus Pull-Down
Modified Curl-Ups
Overhead Press
Triceps Extension
Upper & Lower Body Combined Weightlifting/Resistance Exercises (from past studies)
Calf Raises
Seated Row
Stability Ball (for sit-ups & other exercises) *

Lower Body Weightlifting/Resistance Exercises (from past studies)
Leg Curl
Leg Extension
Leg Press

Note: *Many studies were completed by what I called the notable Australian research team (lead the pack in terms of publications and just nice folks) and some were conducted by the other notable Canadian teams, U.S., and other groups around the world (of course just as nice and wonderful); but overall, this is an area of prostate cancer that surprisingly has received plenty of research for men on ADT thanks to these and other amazing researchers (heck, they deserve Nobel prizes in my mind too)! Of course, more exercises could be added to this table, but this gives the basics of what has already been accomplished. You and your healthcare team may decide to use some of these because they are research-based, or you could construct your own individualized plan.*
*For example, the one exercise I personally added to the table and has not been used in many prostate cancer studies is the stability ball. It allows you to do core workouts, which are critical for strengthening abdominal wall, back and possibly legs without getting on the floor. Getting on the floor with age is not fun, and gets messy, so a stability ball is low-cost and helps target muscles that are often missed (pelvic area) along with other upper and lower body areas when needed, which regardless of your treatment could help with side effects. Hand weights (even resistance bands) can also be purchased and used at home to conduct other versions of the exercises shown in the previous table (if needed), and it allows for a backup plan when someone cannot go to a gym.

CHAPTER 2: BONE-PROTECTING AGENTS (BPAS)

Notes:

CHAPTER 3

Immune Therapies

Provenge and/or other novel biomarker tests to qualify
for additional immune treatments

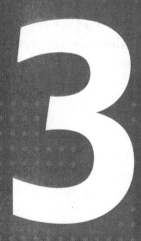

3

PW Quick & Concise Chapter Summary

In general, Provenge provides better potential results when used earlier in CRPC and when PSA is lower. However, biomarker testing can provide access to other immune therapies.

Provenge (also known as "sipuleucel-T") was FDA approved way back in 2010 and became the first personalized immunotherapy for the treatment of prostate cancer to provide a survival benefit for many CRPC patients. In clinical trials, the Provenge group lived significantly longer compared with men in the control group. The Provenge treatment is accomplished by removing a small quantity of your immune cells at a blood bank or medical center. This procedure, which is known as "leukapheresis," takes 2-4 hours ("give some non-boosted immune cells"). Those cells are then sent to one of the company's manufacturing facilities for immune modification or enhancement. After 2-3 days, the patient returns to a doctor's office or medical center trained in this treatment to receive an infusion (IV) of their own ("autologous") boosted immune cells, which takes about an hour and then 30 minutes of monitoring ("get back your boosted immune cells"). This is considered one completed cycle/round, and then this is repeated twice more (cycle or round two and three) and then it is done. So, there is a total of three separate leukapheresis, plus three separate infusion procedures, which equals a total of six appointments over approximately four weeks for patients. In other words, you "give" cells and then "get back" your boosted cells three separate times over a four-week period.

The FDA approved Provenge for men with metastatic CRPC who are without symptoms (asymptomatic) or with minimal symptoms. Basically, if a patient's PSA rises approximately three consecutive times on androgen-deprivation therapy (ADT), and the doctor finds metastatic disease (bone metastasis) using a bone scan or another more sensitive scan/imaging test such as a PET/CT), then that patient qualifies. Based on the phase 3 IMPACT trial, the greatest benefit in terms of improving efficacy and survival with Provenge appears to be when using this option as early as possible, and the lower the PSA the better, as opposed to later when the disease is far more advanced. In addition, despite giving many patients a survival advantage, PSA decreases are not common with this treatment because it appears to be impacting the progression of CRPC using a different method. It has and is being studied now with a variety of CRPC treatments to determine if there is a way to enhance the results even further.

Qualifying for other newer immune therapies, such as pembrolizumab (Keytruda, etc.) is also possible today. However, you typically need to be tested for "biomarkers" to see if you qualify. For example, if you are positive for one of several DNA damage response (DDR) pathways, biomarker tests reflecting DDR, or those which are more common in individuals with DDR (actionable mutations) such as "MSI-H"/dMMR," TMB-H, high PD-L1, etc. then you could work with your medical team to gain access to these other novel immune therapy medicines.

On a separate topic, there are other novel immune treatments that have been getting a lot of attention in some other cancers called "CAR T-cell" therapy. This therapy is now being tested in prostate cancer clinical trials. Finally, please see the PARP inhibitors chapter because these novel therapies also involve biomarker testing to qualify for newer treatments.

Staying on ADT (LHRH, hormone therapy, etc.) is standard practice.

In the clinical trials for Provenge, including the Phase 3 trial resulting in survival benefits and FDA approval, known as the IMPACT study, men stayed on their ADT, so in general it makes sense to do the same. However, that decision will be made in consultation with your medical team. While some believe that hormone therapy gives a slight immune boost itself in the way that it treats the disease, others do not believe this boost exists. Those who believe a boost exists point to an increased immune reaction found at some tumor sites in men who have had their prostate removed and were on ADT before and at the time of surgical removal.

Also, the thymus, a gland in the neck that helps us to mature and perhaps to produce some immune cells, shrinks with age and becomes less functional. However, researchers have noticed in some patients the thymus can begin to grow again and become more active during ADT. Of course, the low testosterone level reached during ADT produces many side effects; but again, it is important to consider that men who were treated in the Provenge phase 3 trial (IMPACT) resulting in FDA approval had castrate levels of testosterone (less than 50 ng/dL or 1.7 nmol/L) during the trial.

An advantage of Provenge is that the treatment is fairly simple, has a low rate of long-term side effects, and gives men another option, before other treatments are used (e.g., androgen receptor or synthesis inhibitors, chemotherapy, etc.). The FDA has also offered flexibility in who can receive it, making it available to men without symptoms or with minimal symptoms of CRPC who have metastatic disease. It is available at certified medical centers and medical offices across the country and both oncologists and urologists can provide Provenge. Interestingly, it is also being tested now in a variety of clinical trial situations from before ADT is even needed (localized disease) to later in the CRPC process.

There is a catch—the treatment is expensive. However, insurance, including Medicare, should cover most of the cost.

Provenge treatment process from start to finish:

Each single round (cycle) is critical, and should not be delayed once the round starts, unless absolutely necessary.

The treatment process with Provenge takes place in three rounds, which are repeated at three different times. You need three rounds or cycles to complete the entire treatment process. In each single round there is a leukapheresis process ("give some non-boosted immune cells"), where blood cells are withdrawn from a patient's arm. The blood goes through a machine that separates some of the white blood cells (immune cells) from the rest of the blood and then collects them. The patient's blood, minus some of those immune cells, is returned to his other arm.

Next, the patient's immune cells are sent to a facility where they are combined with a protein or marker that is unique to prostate cancer cells (prostatic acid phosphatase or PAP). That protein helps produce an immune response to the patient's cancer. Finally, (two to three days after leukapheresis), the immune-activated or boosted cells are returned ("get back your boosted immune cells") via an infusion to the patient to help combat his cancer. So, this now fully completes the first round or cycle. This process is repeated for two additional rounds or cycles, each approximately two weeks apart. Thus, a total of three separate leukapheresis procedures ("give cells") coupled with three separate infusions ("get cells back") of personally activated immune cells at 0, 2, and 4 weeks for a total of six appointments to complete the entire process over a one-month period in the ideal treatment situation. In other words, you "give" cells (leukapheresis) and then "get" back (infusion) your boosted immune cells three different times for a total of six appointments. Put another way, you do the following:

- Give some of your immune cells and then get back your boosted immune cells a few days later (cycle or round one), and then

- Give some more of your immune cells and then get back your boosted cells a few days later (cycle or round two), and then finally

- Give some more of your immune cells and then get back your boosted cells a few days later (cycle or round three), and you have now completed the entire Provenge process in approximately one month!

Provenge is known as an "autologous cellular immunotherapy" treatment because your own immune cells are used, so the donor and recipient are same person (autologous) versus an immune treatment that comes from another person (allogenic). Allogenic treatments are used in some cancers.

Missed or delayed treatment—each round is critical to complete once it has started, but intervals between the three different rounds can be delayed if needed.

Once round one is started, it is important to stay on schedule through the end of round one unless there is a true emergency. If the infusion step (getting back your boosted immune cells) is delayed, then the personalized enhanced cells will not be optimal or usable and the leukapheresis (give cells process) would need to be repeated. The boosting process is really the key treatment step that significantly increases life expectancy in men with CRPC, and you want to receive those boosted cells as soon as they arrive. Any delays in getting back your boosted cells, after giving them, could compromise your results, which is why the entire individual round would need to be repeated to place you in the highest probability of success. In other words, you want your energized or boosted soldiers (enhanced immune cells) to fight the enemy (cancer) when they are working at their peak capacity.

The two-week time interval between an entire round (cycle) is less critical. These can vary if absolutely necessary. Each time one cycle is completed, the patient receives an immune response that lasts for a variable, but lengthy period. The schedule developed is believed to be optimal, but patients appeared to still receive a benefit from a delayed round if the patient's situation called for this delay. Overall, it's best not to delay the scheduled treatments, but your medical team may decide to delay them based on your temporary health, medical, or other personal reasons.

Provenge side effects are mostly temporary, and some can be reduced or prevented by you and your medical team.

The most common side effects that occur within approximately one to two days after each round is completed are (as reported by the New England Journal of Medicine from the IMPACT trial):

- **Chills** (51%)
- **Fever** (23%)
- **Fatigue** (16%)
- **Nausea** (14%)
- **Headache** (11%)

Most of these "flu-like" side effects are temporary and are common with immunotherapies. They are also common with some vaccines, such as the new COVID-19 vaccines. These generally temporary or short-term side effects from Provenge infusions ("getting back your boosted immune cells") typically end within a day or two after the procedure, and some patients are given or recommended acetaminophen and diphenhydramine (also commonly known as "Benadryl" or a generic equivalent) to further reduce these side effects. There were very few cases of dropouts or patients who discontinued the entire treatment because of side effects. In fact, in fewer than 1% of cases were any side effects serious enough to stop a patient from receiving all three infusions (getting back your boosted immune cells). There were also no differences in safety between older and younger men. Men who were included in the IMPACT trial ranged from 40 to over 90 years of age, with a median age of 71 years (half the participants were below and half of them were above age 71).

PSA does not have to change or decrease to get a benefit, but again lower PSA is usually better when receiving Provenge.

Since this treatment works in a different way, it is worth considering how medical teams know whether patients are responding to Provenge. There is only a drop in PSA or change in an imaging test, such as a bone scan (newer more sensitive PET/CT scans may or may not see something different) in a minority of patients. The FDA no longer bases its evaluation of response in clinical trials for men with CRPC on a change in PSA, but rather on an extension of life. The FDA evaluation change makes a great deal of sense since these therapies may not change PSA but can still extend life or improve prognosis. This is what was demonstrated in Provenge clinical trials. Provenge extended survival in patients with CRPC significantly more than the control group and therefore was approved by the FDA for treating some CRPC patients.

Again, the good news about Provenge is ideally it takes just four weeks to complete the entire treatment process, which suggests you and your healthcare team should already have a plan in place before, during, or right after these treatments to decide what other cancer fighting medications (if any) should be added to your current or future treatment plan. Remember, the lower the PSA and the earlier in the course of metastatic CRPC then the higher probability of positive results with Provenge. Immunotherapy in this specific case with Provenge tends to work better in many patients when their immune system is still working well, and the tumor burden is lower. Although, in other cases or with newer immune cancer drugs they may work much better in people positive for certain or specific biomarker tests (more on this later in the chapter).

Life extension in months is misunderstood.

Another issue that needs to be resolved is the 4.1-month survival benefit specifically cited with Provenge from the IMPACT trial by many sources, as well as any other specific month or years of survival mentioned, or not mentioned, for other approved drugs in this book. The initial reaction by many is to assume 4.1 months is not much, which is completely understandable. However, a closer look at this or any other FDA approved treatment for CRPC suggests something very different for many patients. In the IMPACT trial, half the patients taking Provenge survived longer than the 4.1-month time period and half shorter. About a third of the men were still alive three years after treatment! Also, these were the results before and during 2010, which was before the majority of other medicines in this book were approved. There has been a new drug approved to be used with or after Provenge approximately every year or two since this immune therapy was introduced, and these other medications can also improve survival, which only adds to a greater or more positive CRPC prognosis.

In other words, the survival or extension of life keeps getting longer, so a CRPC drug that improves survival today should only fuel optimism of better responses or higher expectations (not lower). These achievements also allow for the study of novel combinations of drugs or treatments, which could provide a response far greater than any drug used alone. The take home message is that the survival period in months does not adequately reflect the reality of the benefits observed today. It is part of the reason future predictions of prostate cancer survival continue to be one of the most optimistic compared to almost any other adult cancer!

Provenge before, after, or with other treatments—but before or earlier still appears better.

Approximately 20% of the men from the IMPACT phase 3 trial had already received chemotherapy when they were treated with Provenge, so it would be expected that some chemotherapy patients would also qualify for Provenge. Still, an interesting analysis found that men seemed to have significantly prolonged their lives on chemotherapy (e.g., Taxotere or docetaxel) if they had received Provenge before the chemotherapy. Thus, it seems Provenge may have improved the efficacy of a later treatment. Again, this is part of the reason the earlier use of Provenge in the metastatic asymptomatic or minimally symptomatic CRPC process, the better the chance of success.

Additionally, preliminary clinical trials suggest using Provenge with certain anti-androgen receptor or synthesis inhibitors (ARIs or ASIs) is not only an option but had no negative impact on the effectiveness of Provenge and, overall, has a good safety profile. Therefore, it should be part of your treatment discussion with your medical team.

In the Provenge IMPACT clinical study, almost half (48%) of the men were also on bone-protection agents (BPAs) when the study started, which means Provenge can be used in men whether they are taking these medications or not.

Interestingly, Provenge is even being tested with Xofigo and other treatments for earlier stage bone predominant, minimally symptomatic CRPC to see if an even greater effect could be achieved. This makes a lot of sense, and so we are hopeful one or more of these combinations will be used soon.

Provenge is still a CRPC option if cancer is in the lymph nodes only and not in the bones.

Since a small percentage of men with CRPC in the Provenge clinical trials had cancer only in their lymph nodes, insurance could cover men in this situation, allowing them to receive Provenge. However, there are many men with prostate cancer who have cancer in their lymph nodes and are still sensitive to androgen-suppression therapy and/or radiation. These men do not have CRPC, which means they would not be eligible to receive Provenge at this time.

PW Lifestyle Empowerment Moment

One of the most important parts of the Provenge process involves lifestyle changes, which does not get enough attention! First, being well-hydrated before the leukapheresis ("give some non-boosted cells") procedure is extremely important and should be emphasized to every patient. It is critical to consume enough water to cause your urine to be almost clear in color, which usually reflects a person that is well hydrated compared to a moderate or darker yellow urine color that could be a sign that you are dehydrated, or not well-hydrated. Dehydration can cause the procedure to take much longer, and in rare cases has delayed or interrupted treatment. It can cause clumping of cells or blockage of the tubing connected to the leukapheresis machine, so that cell extraction is not as efficient. This is why we like to say: "hydration prevents Provenge interruptions," or "H2O allows Provenge to go," or "without some water the first step of the Provenge process could be a non-starter." I think you get the idea here. Hydration allows for the components of the blood to flow smoothly through the tubes being used and reduces the risk of that so-called "clogging effect." When it comes to fluid intake, please remember the saying "clear is cool," which again essentially means being fully hydrated (not overhydrated, which could require a sudden urge for a portable urinal device) is really one of the most important things you can do.

In addition, it is always worth considering other lifestyle factors, such as diet or even dietary supplements when undergoing Provenge treatment. Generally speaking, "less is more" during this treatment when it comes to dietary supplements. Provenge patients should ideally not take any supplement that says it is an "immune booster," "immune modulator," or that makes any claims to "support immune health" or "support the immune system." Not only were these supplements not studied in conjunction with Provenge treatment, but theoretically such supplements could block or disrupt the action of Provenge, or even encourage an autoimmune reaction. No one knows currently, but why risk a proven therapy with something unproven in combination with this therapy? In other words, it's better to be safe than risk not being safe. If a new study comes along suggesting otherwise then this could change things, but this has not occurred thus far.

However, there is an exception in the supplement world with Provenge that you should discuss with your medical team. There is another temporary condition associated with Provenge known as a "paresthesia," which is a sensation of tingling, prickling, or numbness of the skin around the mouth. The feeling is similar to the feeling one gets when a part of the body temporarily falls asleep. There are many causes of paresthesia, and one of them can be the leukapheresis procedure itself. During the process, a citrate compound (in addition to the water you consume as mentioned earlier), is used to prevent components of the blood from sticking together as a patient's immune cells are collected. However, citrate can temporarily bind to calcium in your blood and lower the level of free calcium, causing this hypersensitive nerve reaction (paresthesia). While it generally causes no long-term problems, paresthesia can make it difficult for patients to recover from a treatment or receive another treatment. You might be able to prevent it or reduce the risk by working with your medical team and taking a calcium carbonate dietary supplement. This is the one exception to the previous discussion of less is more when it comes to dietary supplements and Provenge.

In fact, several small studies have demonstrated that taking a calcium carbonate dietary supplement (1000-1500 mg/day from studies—but dosage should be decided by your medical team) around the time of the leukapheresis procedure may reduce the risk of paresthesia by supplying the blood with more calcium. This is also good potential advice for many men with CRPC in general because bone loss and hypocalcemia is a concern, as mentioned in the last chapter on bone protecting agents (BPAs). However, taking calcium in the form of calcium carbonate is key because calcium citrate supplements could theoretically increase the risk of paresthesia or make it worse, because citrate used in the leukapheresis procedure itself appears to increase the risk, so why voluntarily add more than is necessary? Instead, taking 1000-1200 mg of calcium carbonate daily, for example, the day before, the day of, and for a week after each of the three separate leukapheresis procedures may prevent or reduce this side effect. Talk to your medical team about making this change or the latest protocol to help reduce the risk of paresthesia after leukapheresis. Calcium carbonate chews or powder (not pills) in a variety of flavors and forms (e.g., TUMS, Rolaids, or generic brands) are even easier to take and you can bring them with you the day of the procedure just in case your doctor thinks you need more calcium right after the procedure because of this potential temporary, but still annoying side effect. So, remember when it comes to the leukapheresis **"CLEAR IS COOL"** and **"CALCIUM CARBONATE COULD BE COOL, TOO."**

In terms of other lifestyle tips, what is generally good for your heart is good for your immune system. Heart Healthy = Immune Healthy! If you think about all the things in life that are heart healthy, almost all of them help make your immune system as healthy as possible. A healthy weight/waist, blood cholesterol, blood pressure and blood sugar, along with a better diet, better sleep quality or quantity, and exercise or physical activity is overall heart and immune healthy. It is also heart and immune healthy to be caught up on all your adult vaccinations (e.g., Covid, flu, pneumonia, shingles, tetanus, etc.), which was also covered in the first chapter. Please first ask your medical team which adult preventive vaccines you are and are not able to get or catch up on right now or in the future.

"Tissue Agnostics" or getting a drug for any cancer type based primarily on biomarker testing

New immune therapies are potentially accessible, but you need to work with your medical team and determine when to be tested for these biomarkers to see if you qualify.

Something quite remarkable has happened recently in prostate and many other cancer treatments. Since the last edition of this book, just a few years ago, drugs were only approved for specific cancers based on studies of those specific drugs working only against those specific cancers, as is the case for most of the drugs in this book. However, what is remarkable is that approval groups such as the FDA are beginning to approve some drugs, including newer immune therapies, based on the principle of "tissue agnostics." Another definition of the word "agnostic" means noncommittal or not preferential. This means that regardless of the cancer or solid tumor type, if your biomarker test comes up positive then you qualify for a potential beneficial drug!

Today, there are numerous immune therapies approved for different types of cancer. Many cancers may ultimately express biomarker or molecular changes that, if detected, may increase the chances that you can respond to one of these newer immune therapy drugs. Therefore, the FDA approved the potential access of these newer medications, such as pembrolizumab (Keytruda) if you are tested and positive for what is known as "Microsatellite Instability-High (MSI-H)" or "Mismatch Repair Deficient (dMMR)," or a "Tumor Mutational Burden-High (TMB-H) with approximately equal to or greater than 10 mutations/megabase (mut/Mb)" prostate cancer, as determined by an FDA-approved test. It is also more common to qualify for this immune therapy when your cancer has "progressed following prior treatment and there are no satisfactory alternative treatment options" (from Keytruda prescribing information and the FDA).

For example, if a cancer has a large or high number of genetic mutations from biomarker or tumor genetic testing (TMB-H) then you could qualify. Also, if a cancer contains certain genetic changes that impact a cell's ability to repair injured or damaged DNA, then this is essentially what is known as MSI-H tumors, or in many cases can be known as dMMR. There is an association between MSI-H and TMB-H since many MSI-H cancers also can have TMB-H. However, many TMB-H tumors are not associated with MSI-H, so it is not vice versa, which is why these specific tissue or blood tests are so critical at a time when someone is looking for a new treatment for their cancer. TMB-H is more common than MSI-H, so again the importance of testing. In fact, many patients must still be tested for these molecular alterations or biomarkers to officially qualify for these newer options. Still, just because someone tests positive for these unique tests does not guarantee a response to this or a similar immune therapy. However, it first officially qualifies you for receiving it, and second, it increases the probability that you could have a positive response.

Why give these newer immune drugs only when one of the above or other tests are positive? Cancer cells that are positive for these or other novel tests (DNA damage repair—DDR such as BRCA-1/2, defective mismatch repair-dMMR, high inflammatory infiltrate levels, etc.), or other so-called "immunogenic signatures" in many cases will display a large number of mutated proteins on the surface of their cells. These proteins make it harder for the cells to hide from the immune system and are more likely to attract the immune system toward the cancer, especially when given an immune boost from these various therapies. Drugs such as Keytruda (pembrolizumab), and others such as Opdivo (nivolumab) and Yervoy (ipilimumab), Tecentriq (atezolizumab), etc. are now being tested in a variety of situations along with determining which immunogenic signatures or biomarkers are the very best to qualify for these therapies. In some (not all) of these clinical trials PSA was also being reduced with some immune treatments, while also demonstrating a prognostic benefit.

The take home message needs to be reiterated because we could have written a book just on this subject: If you are positive for one of several DNA damage response (DDR) pathways, biomarker tests reflecting DDR, or which are more common in individuals with DDR (actionable mutations) such as "MSI-H"/ dMMR," TMB-H, high PD-L1, etc., then you could work with your medical team to gain access to these other novel immune therapy medications.

CAR T-cell/gene therapy

T-cells genetically engineered to attack a specific protein found on the cancer cell surface and even CAR NK cells.

It seems there are endless clinical studies of similar and different immune drugs being tested with various other therapies, as mentioned in the previous section. One special type of immune treatment that has dramatically changed the course of some types or forms of leukemia, lymphoma, and now multiple myeloma is called "Chimeric Antigen Receptor (CAR) T-cell therapy." The incredible process usually goes as follows:

Step 1: T-cells (a type of immune cell) are collected from the blood of a patient (leukapheresis or apheresis).

Step 2: In the laboratory, gene therapy is used by taking the gene of a specialized receptor (CAR) and inserting into those T-cells, and then millions to billions of these special CAR T-cells are grown in the lab.

Step 3: CAR T-cells, or these genetically engineered T-cells produced in the lab are now given back or infused into the same patient after they have received several days of low-dose immune suppressive therapy (also sometimes referred to as a conditioning chemotherapy regimen) to prepare their body to receive the CAR T-cells, and not unfavorably react to them creating an auto-immune situation. Then these CAR T-cells can recognize or bind to those specific proteins on cancer cells and eliminate them.

Again, the good news for certain blood (hematologic) cancers is it has completely changed treatment and put many patients into remission. It usually only requires a one-time infusion of the CAR T-cells and responses can occur quite quickly in other cancers. And now for the catch—apart from the enormous price tag associated with these therapies, and the potential for very serious and life-threatening side effects that need to be monitored, is the additional fact that solid tumors (not blood cancers) such as prostate cancer are having a tough time getting most patients to respond to newer immune therapies, in general. Perhaps because there are many obstacles getting in the way of reaching these types of cancer cells, and because prostate cancer is often not associated with a lot of mutations (aka low mutational burden) unless a cancer has more unique or aggressive features. However, this could just be a time or learning curve issue because researchers are constantly looking for the right markers to predict response to immune drugs, and in the right situations, for example, before, during, or after chemotherapy, radiation and other treatments.

CAR T-cell therapy holds a potential advantage because it involves essentially laboratory produced or synthetic molecules able to recognize intact proteins in the body without the need of overcoming other known obstacles of other immune therapies. However, will it work, and will it work soon? CAR-T for prostate cancer currently has multiple clinical trials in the U.S. and all over the world. Whether it is a future option is another part of the immune therapy discussion with your medical team.

The purpose of this chapter was to show you the exciting diverse immune therapies available right now and possibly very soon in prostate cancer. These therapies, coming from multiple directions, should provide enormous optimism. It is easy to forget about the various immune products made in our bodies, such as antibodies, T-cells and other types of immune compounds that destroy bacteria, viruses, fungi, and other invaders throughout our life, and patrol areas of the body to prevent cancer initiation and growth during our childhood and many of our adult years. If we can sensitize our immune system's ability to protect us, as it did in many of us during our younger years, then treatment possibilities also abound!

Again, immune therapy is not just one category of treatment, but consists of endless diverse possibilities to exploit the vulnerabilities of many tumor types. In fact, at the time of this book publication, even different types of CAR immune cell therapies are being explored against prostate and other cancers, including CAR NK (Natural Killer Cells), which is another part of the immune system able to destroy cancer cells directly. But these can come from many outside sources (not just the patient) and should also be less expensive and less toxic. The list of potential opportunities seems endless!

Biomarker testing is needed to qualify for PARP Inhibitors.

(For a more comprehensive discussion on this topic, please see the chapter on PARP inhibitors.) PARP inhibitors are pills for patients dealing with potentially more aggressive prostate cancer based on results of biomarker tests, such as the ones described earlier, especially BRCA-1/2 (DDR) and other results. In other words, patients today can qualify not only for immune therapies with these biomarker tests, but also pills that do not allow specific cancers to repair themselves or replicate when they are damaged!

Notes:

_____

_____

_____

_____

_____

_____

_____

_____

_____

_____

_____

_____

_____

_____

_____

_____

CHAPTER 4

ARIs or ASIs

Androgen Receptor Inhibitors (ARIs): Erleada, Nubeqa, Xtandi or Androgen Synthesis Inhibitors (ASI): Zytiga (abiraterone) and Yonsa (abiraterone)

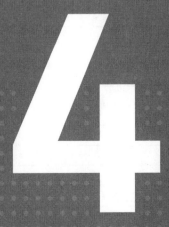

PW Quick & Concise Chapter Message

Here is another part of the book which could be helpful for some men who do not have CRPC, but rather metastatic castration-sensitive prostate cancer (mCSPC). These are men whose testosterone is below 50 ng/dL (1.7 nmol/L) and are still PSA responsive to traditional ADT (hormone sensitive cancer). More specifically, the cancer has spread beyond the prostate, or where the prostate used to be, and there is now at least one cancer lesion on a bone and, in some cases, also in more distant lymph nodes or an organ. But again, the cancer is still very responsive to ADT. So, why not just use ADT alone? It was found that adding one of these types of pills (ARI or ASI) in this situation along with ADT worked much better than ADT alone!

Chemotherapy has also been found to be helpful for some men with mCSPC. Additionally, the pills described in this chapter are also FDA approved and work against different types of CRPC! Therefore, this chapter is also for some men with two different forms of CRPC, which are known as "non-metastatic CRPC (nmCRPC)" and "metastatic CRPC (mCRPC)." In other words, when the cancer is aggressive then using these options earlier in the process may provide better results, which is part of the reason they were approved. Yes!

Some of these pills helped men with mCRPC and then were tried with men earlier in the prostate cancer process, where they also worked in slowing progression or improving survival. Please keep in mind if any of these medications used along with ADT are no longer working, or become less effective, your medical team will discuss what the next steps should be regarding treatment. This is where the treatments discussed in other chapters of this book become even more important.

Currently, there are three forms or types of prostate cancer where one or more of the ARI drugs are approved and two situations where an ASI is approved. These prostate cancer situations are as follows:

- **Metastatic castration-sensitive prostate cancer** (mCSPC)
- **Non-metastatic CRPC** (nmCRPC)
- **Metastatic castration-resistant prostate cancer** (mCRPC)

At the time this book was published the following drugs were approved for these types of prostate cancer:

- **Erleada** (also known as "apalutamide") is approved currently for mCSPC, and nmCRPC.
- **Nubeqa** (also known as "darolutamide") is approved for nmCRPC.
- **Xtandi** (also known as "enzalutamide") is approved for mCSPC, nmCRPC, and mCRPC.
- **Zytiga** (also known as "abiraterone") is approved for mCSPC, and mCRPC.

Note: *There is also a pill known as "Yonsa," and it has the same active ingredient (abiraterone) as Zytiga, but it has enhanced bioavailability and is usually given in a lower (50% less) dose than Zytiga. It can be taken with or without food, while Zytiga must be taken without food—at least two hours before or one hour after a meal. Yonsa is also specifically approved for mCRPC. All abiraterone pills, whether its Zytiga or Yonsa, should be swallowed whole with water.*

The name(s) of the phase 3 trials, which allowed these drugs to be approved and/or at least provided some of the best information in terms of their efficacy and safety, are in parentheses and quotations ("...") next to the type of prostate cancer they are indicated to treat:

- **Erleada** for mCSPC ("TITAN") and nmCRPC ("SPARTAN")
- **Nubeqa** for nmCRPC ("ARAMIS")

- **Xtandi** for mCSPC ("ARCHES" & "ENZAMET"),
  nmCRPC ("PROSPER"),
  mCRPC ("AFFIRM" & "PREVAIL")
- **Zytiga** for mCSPC ("LATITUDE" & "STAMPEDE"),
  and mCRPC ("AA-COU-301, and "AA-COU-302").

Note: *As mentioned above there is now another drug known as "Yonsa," which is a micronized/fine particle form of abiraterone—the same active ingredient as Zytiga. However, Yonsa has a different manufacturer and can be given in a lower dosage with or without food versus Zytiga (without food only). Yonsa (along with daily methylprednisolone) was approved as an alternative abiraterone option for mCRPC based on the phase 2 STARR clinical study and the fact that abiraterone already had two successful phase 3 trials mentioned above ("AA-COU-301," and "AA-COU-302").*

When discussing this information with your medical team, it may be helpful to put it in table form, including what the situation looks like right now, with current medication, along with the types of prostate cancer these medications could be used for at the present time (see below). We also always try to include the official abbreviated name of the phase 3 clinical trial(s) that helped the drug either get FDA approved or another phase 3 trial that helped in better understanding the efficacy and safety of the drug. A search on the internet using the official name of the phase 3 trial allows you access to the methods and often updated results of each trial. In fact, most of the phase 3 trials' original, updated medical publications, and even many editorials or reviews of these studies are also available at no charge and can be located again by searching the name of the study. We understand it can be overwhelming at times to keep track of all the names of drugs and trials covered in this chapter, but we feel it is necessary to provide patients with all the information they need to make good decisions along with your medical team. In this chapter, we also added one phase-2 trial because it helped an alternative form of Zytiga, known as Yonsa, get FDA approved.

Additionally, phase 3 clinical trial names could also help improve communication and understanding between you and your medical team to get a better idea of what to potentially expect in terms of efficacy and side effects. Therefore, when talking about progression or survival or any other clinical findings, including mild-to-severe side effects, it is helpful to refer to the phase 3 trial names in your discussion. Again, the trial results are also fairly easy to find using an internet search. Your medical team has ongoing experience with some or many of these medications, which should be discussed because they can provide the most recent and relevant ground-breaking research (benefits and side effects).

mCSPC	nmCRPC	mCRPC
metastatic castration-sensitive prostate cancer FDA approved drugs (phase 3 trial abbreviated names)	non-metastatic castration-resistant prostate cancer FDA approved drugs (phase 3 trial abbreviated names)	metastatic castration-resistant prostate cancer FDA approved drugs (phase 3 trial abbreviated names)
Erleada (TITAN phase 3)	**Erleada** (SPARTAN phase 3)	**Xtandi** (AFFIRM phase 3 after chemotherapy and PREVAIL phase 3 before chemotherapy)
Xtandi (ARCHES phase 3) (ENZAMET phase 3)	**Nubeqa** (ARAMIS phase 3)	**Yonsa with daily methylprednisolone** (STARR phase 2)—alternative lower dose form—with or without food form of abiraterone/Zytiga
Zytiga with daily prednisone (LATITUDE phase 3) (STAMPEDE phase 3)	**Xtandi** (PROSPER phase 3)	**Zytiga with daily prednisone** (AA-COU-301 phase 3 after chemotherapy and AA-COU-302 phase 3 before chemotherapy

Note: *In the mCRPC studies above where the drugs Xtandi (AFFIRM trial) or Zytiga (AA-COU-301 trial) were used after chemotherapy, in general, the chemotherapy drug that was utilized before trying Xtandi or Zytiga was Taxotere (docetaxel).*

Once you qualify for one of these treatments, the similar and unique side effects of each should be a major part of discussions with your medical team. All of these are pill treatments, and some can be taken with or without food (Erleada, Xtandi, Yonsa), while others must be taken with food (Nubeqa), and one (Zytiga) should only be taken with water on an empty stomach—without food at least two hours before or one hour after a meal.

Also noteworthy is a recent phase 3 clinical trial of men with mCRPC that had not received chemotherapy called "ACIS." In the ACIS trial, men with mCRPC were placed on Erleada and Zytiga together (combination) versus Zytiga only. Although the combination appeared to slow the progression of cancer, the trial was halted because it did not appear to impact overall survival. This study and additional findings coming from it should be discussed with your healthcare team. Regardless, it appears the use of an ARI and then an ASI, or vice versa, after no longer responding to one or the other has provided limited or minimal, if any, benefit. But again, please discuss this research with your healthcare team because all these situations in prostate cancer have exceptions, or the need for further personal clarifications, which are better than this book can provide or explain.

Note: *It is easy to get caught up in what we term "micro-analysis," where each drug is compared or analyzed based on every finding. This is another of the many reasons your medical team is so valuable because they can walk you through the findings or side effects they consider "clinically valuable" versus those that are more "clinically trivial" based on their knowledge and experience, as well as working with you personally and understanding your preferences or options as an individual (not just an "average" statistical data point).*

There are now three androgen receptor inhibitors (ARIs) and two androgen synthesis inhibitors (ASIs)—

oral drugs available and/choosing which one is right for you should be personalized with your medical team based on your type of prostate cancer (mCSPC, nmCRPC, mCRPC, etc.), if you qualify. They are all effective for many reasons and part of their difference may depend on the different side effects of each.

Few other innovations in prostate cancer research exemplify the ongoing progress in treatments better than the androgen receptor inhibitors (ARIs) or androgen synthesis inhibitors (ASIs). The ARIs are also referred to as nonsteroidal anti-androgens, or even "second generation anti-androgens" or "second-generation androgen receptor antagonists," since they block the binding of androgens (such as testosterone) to the cancer cell's androgen receptor (AR). In fact, they fit much tighter into that receptor, and do not stimulate it, compared to the older (first generation) anti-androgen drugs. Yet, before these drugs were invented many believed ADT, by reducing testosterone to below 50 ng/dL (1.7 nmol/L), was enough to eliminate all the available precursors to testosterone and testosterone itself from stimulating a prostate tumor. The older concept of using first generation anti-androgen pills with ADT was believed to be enough to reduce or stop androgens from stimulating tumors, which turned out not to be effective enough for some situations. Even the small amount of detectable testosterone in the body, or precursors of testosterone coming from other organs (like the adrenal gland on top of the kidneys) can still fuel many prostate cancers.

In fact, it is now well-known that some prostate cancers can essentially make their own testosterone when there is little or none left in the body, so they can fuel themselves. However, they need, rely, and simply depend on that AR to keep functioning. It was this interesting discovery that CRPC is not completely insensitive to androgens or hormones, that led to the older term HRPC ("hormone" refractory prostate cancer), or AIPC ("androgen" independent prostate cancer) to become outdated. Therefore, the term CRPC became the leading name for when a prostate cancer no longer responds to ADT.

In short, a rising PSA, despite castrate levels of testosterone, is what is known today as "CRPC." That definition or abbreviation allows for the possibility that other androgens from the body, or from the tumor itself, are still able to provide some fuel for the cancer and can still be impacted by "hormones" or "androgens." Since the cancer is not completely hormone refractory or completely androgen independent, CRPC has become the widely accepted term for a prostate cancer no longer responding to traditional ADT.

To make this clearer, and further demonstrate the power of these drugs, think of androgens (testosterone and other hormones) as potential fuel sources for a cancer. However, they cannot act as an actual fuel source unless they reach the inside of the cancer cell to then fuel the internal workings, or machinery of the cell. It is like a fuel door cover with a lock on it that does not allow fuel to reach the tank of a difficult to control car, which needs to run out of gas to stop moving, unless there is a key or switch to open the fuel door. So, how does the fuel get inside the cell when the outside has that locked fuel door or cover?

The outside of a cancer cell has locks, or androgen receptors (AR), but when androgens (keys) reach the AR (lock) then essentially the AR goes from locked to unlocked, which now allows the androgens (fuel) to reach the inside. When fuel/signals from the outside reach the inside of the machine or actual internal tank it can then help feed the engine and rest of the car to keep it moving, functional and driving erratically. In other words, it allows the tumor to grow, survive, thrive and even replicate. Therefore, stopping the key from being produced (lowering or eliminating androgens) or from fitting into the lock (AR) should be one of the goals in making treatment more effective. All these ARI drugs have a somewhat similar mechanism of action because they "block the lock" (AR) and the ability of the key (androgens) to fit into the lock (AR). Preventing the key from fitting into the lock keeps the door closed, again preventing fuel sources from reaching the tumor, which would otherwise allow it to grow, replicate, or cause more damage.

These newer second-generation ARI drugs also work well beyond what goes on with the lock and key example. Unlike the older first-generation anti-androgen pills (bicalutamide, which was also known as "casodex," flutamide, nilutamide, etc.) used with ADT, these newer drugs can cause multiple things to happen, which makes them so effective, including:

- Blocks or inhibits the ability of the AR to be translocated or brought deep within a cell, which would usually send a more direct message to the cancer cell, for example to grow.

- Blocks or inhibits DNA binding, so a signal, even if it gets through, cannot be adequately translated to or used by the cancer cells.

- Blocks or inhibits the ability to stimulate the AR partially or even minimally, which some of the older first-generation drugs did in certain cases—they had some "agonist" activity.

All these newer ARI drugs block or inhibit multiple steps, which is why they are so effective. They not only help stop cancer growth, but in many cases, they can also help shrink and eliminate some tumors. So, why not use them (or ASI drugs) with ADT before CRPC occurs, particularly in certain men with high-risk or metastatic CSPC (castration sensitive prostate cancer)? This is exactly what is happening now. These drugs are being used before CRPC occurs for some aggressive prostate cancers, and when combined with traditional ADT they are demonstrating some remarkable results, along with some unique side effects.

Androgen Synthesis Inhibitors (ASIs)—

Zytiga and Yonsa both contain the active ingredient abiraterone, but Zytiga is approved for mCRPC and metastatic high-risk CSPC (mCSPC) and is taken with daily prednisone. Yonsa is approved for mCRPC and is taken with daily

methylprednisolone. Zytiga should be taken on an empty stomach with water at least two hours before or one hour after a meal. Yonsa is a micronized pill allowing for a lower daily dose of abiraterone with or without food.

Zytiga (also known as "abiraterone") is an androgen synthesis inhibitor (ASI), or sometimes also called an androgen biosynthesis inhibitor, or "second-generation" or "selective" ASI because there was another ASI used in the past known as "ketoconazole," which has a less selective/targeted impact on the enzyme important for the synthesis of androgens. However, rather than blocking the key from fitting into the lock from our last example with ARIs, Zytiga simply reduces the production of the keys (androgens) from the three primary locations where androgens are produced, which include:

- Testicles (location where ADT also helps)
- Adrenal glands
- Cancer itself

In this case, it is not about blocking a lock from a fuel source, but rather not allowing the fuel source (or key) itself to be created in the first place. Although it uses a different route, the goal is similar, which is not providing a fuel source to a difficult to control car, allowing it to be slowed down by running out of gas, and thus stopping it from causing more damage.

Zytiga (abiraterone) is FDA approved for high-risk Castration Sensitive Prostate Cancer (CSPC), and for CRPC either before or after chemotherapy. Prednisone is also given with daily Zytiga to reduce some of the more serious potential side effects of this drug, which is why it is so important to take the combination.

Additionally, there is another abiraterone product available on the market known as "Yonsa," which uses the same active ingredient as Zytiga or abiraterone, but it is a "micronized" or "fine-particle" version of it in a tablet/pill form. This means it has an increased surface area, which allows for a reduced particle size, allowing better absorption. Again, it is the same active ingredient (abiraterone acetate), but it is used with 4 mg of daily methylprednisolone, which is in the same drug class (glucocorticoids or corticosteroids) as prednisone. In fact, 4 mg of methylprednisolone is essentially equivalent to 5 mg of prednisone in terms of strength. Yonsa comes in a smaller dose (125 mg tablets—total daily dosage of 500 mg) and is similar in efficacy compared to Zytiga (250 tablets—total daily dosage of 1000 mg). Yonsa can be taken with or without food, whereas Zytiga needs to be taken without food. Yonsa was approved for mCRPC based on a phase 2 study known as STARR, but Zytiga is approved for CSPC and mCRPC (before or after chemotherapy—two separate phase 3 trials—AA-COU-301 and AA-COU-302).

No book should decide which ARI or ASI is personally best for you—

but this section could help facilitate the discussion with your healthcare team about the catches and side effects.

First, we will introduce these drugs in alphabetical order by their commercial or trade names, along with their generic names (in the parentheses), which makes them easier to discuss and memorize. Also, their respective websites are provided, because in our opinion the large number of options, ongoing additional approvals, and some of the most updated information on new treatment effects or indications and side effects are found there. The websites also help guide patients to additional financial, insurance or lack of insurance questions.

- **Erleada** (also known as "apalutamide")—**erleada.com**
- **Nubeqa** (also known as "darolutamide")—**nubeqa.com**
- **Xtandi** (also known as "enzalutamide")—**xtandi.com**
- **Zytiga/Yonsa** (also known as "abiraterone")—**zytiga.com** or **yonsarx.com**

All the above ARI pills are approved for "nmCRPC" or non-metastatic CRPC (also known as "M0 CRPC"). Erleada or

Zytiga are also approved for mCSPC (metastatic Castration Sensitive Prostate Cancer), which means the cancer is generally still primarily sensitive to androgens and PSA remains low while the testosterone is low. Xtandi is also approved for mCSPC, as well as mCRPC, and Zytiga/Yonsa is approved for mCRPC.

Again, the focus of discussions with your medical team should be on whether any of these pills are right for you, and if so, which one specifically is appropriate for you based on your individual situation. Because the similar and unique side effects of each one is also important, we will do a quick review of the type or form of prostate cancer and each drug indicated (ARI or ASI) for that form in terms of quick benefits and side effects.

PW Lifestyle Empowerment Moment

- Taking medication as directed is very important.
- Erleada or Xtandi or Yonsa can be taken with or without food.
- Nubeqa should be taken with food.
- Zytiga should be taken on an empty stomach—without food at least two hours before or one hour after a meal.

PW Lifestyle Empowerment Moment

It is interesting that the global popularity of CBD (cannabidiol), either over the counter (OTC) or as a prescription has not initiated enough studies to derive a definitive conclusion as to how these newer or older prostate cancer pills (including the ARIs or ASIs, as well as the PARP inhibitor drugs from chapter 7) are more specifically and metabolically impacted by CBD (good, bad, or indifferent). CBD is a strong inhibitor of some metabolic or detoxifying enzymes in the liver that could theoretically increase the exposure to other drugs, as well as the side effects from them. Additionally, CBD and other cannabinoid medications (marijuana or derivatives from it, etc.) could have their metabolism increased, so there is less exposure or efficacy, or some drugs could theoretically decrease their metabolism/breakdown, so there is more exposure to CBD, and increased risk of side effects.

In short, there is no definitive answer to the questions concerning the impact of CBD on these prostate cancer pills, so you should just be aware of this issue. Ask your medical team about the latest drug interaction studies of the ARIs and ASIs, especially if you are considering using any of them, or even CBD. As an example, ketoconazole, an older non-selective ASI, was found to increase concentrations of THC (delta-9-tetrahydrocannabinol), which is a primary cannabinoid found in marijuana, and increase CBD concentrations from a past study. CBD is known to cause an increased exposure to other non-prostate cancer drugs, which could increase the toxicity of those medications. So, it would be nice to know these answers.

One of the only prescription CBD medications is called "Epidiolex" and was approved by the FDA for the treatment of seizures associated with certain rare syndromes in patients one year of age and older. The reason we mention "Epidiolex" is the fact that it has undergone some of the more methodologically rigorous studies to determine side effects. So, it is important to continue to follow any adverse (or positive) effects of this drug and relate it to what could be observed with CBD. Additionally, this company is testing purified forms of CBD and THC in other medical situations, so looking for additional education from their studies is of great interest.

There is also strong interest in whether cannabinoids such as THC or CBD can fight cancer because there have been cannabinoid receptors found on some prostate cancer cells. However, the reality is there is no methodologically strong data to suggest these compounds could help, harm, or do anything against prostate cancer. With hundreds of ongoing clinical trials, it makes sense to check with your healthcare team regarding the research on this subject because it could quickly change in the positive or negative direction.

Currently, the biggest interest and potential application for THC and/or CBD within cancer is to reduce some potential side effects of conventional treatments. This discussion should be handled by your medical team to determine if there are any such adverse effects they believe could be alleviated. For example, Marinol (dronabinol in a pill) or Syndros (another dronabinol product but in liquid form), both contain a synthetic form of THC and have been FDA approved to reduce chemotherapy-induced nausea and vomiting (CINV) "in patients who have failed to respond adequately to conventional antiemetic treatments." Cesamet (nabilone) is another synthetic cannabinoid (like THC), which has a similar indication as Marinol and Syndros. There has been tremendous recent excitement for CBD and marijuana in treating certain conditions or side effects, but some people do not realize the first prescription laboratory created cannabinoid, Marinol, has been available in cancer for the treatment of CINV since 1985! In other words, despite the recent surge in interest, medicine and medical research have been using derivatives of marijuana for some time in cancer. The downside is the lack of clear understanding of their interactions or effects (good or bad) with today's well-proven prostate cancer treatments. And, again, you know what we are going to say by now...this is where a discussion with your medical team is better than this book.

mCSPC, nmCRPC, and mCRPC

Starting on the next page, we will again mention the drugs approved for mCSPC, nmCRPC, and mCRPC, and briefly mention some of the treatment benefits. Finally, we will spend the rest of the chapter on common and not so common side effects of each drug. All of this will help facilitate your conversations with your medical team. Keep in mind, men were also on traditional ADT (GnRH, LHRH injections, etc.) in addition to these newer pills.

Metastatic castration-sensitive prostate cancer (mCSPC)

Note: Erleada, Xtandi and Zytiga are individually FDA approved for patients with mCSPC

Important treatment note: Rather than micro-dissecting all the different treatment benefits and clinical trials, which could be another book, the generalized benefits of these approved drugs were for some or all the following:

- Improving or favorably impacting "overall survival" or living longer when on one of these medications + ADT was compared to the placebo or control group + ADT.

- Reducing the risk of prostate cancer progressing or spreading further in the body. This is also known in some situations as improving "radiographic progression-free survival" (rPFS).

- Delaying the time in needing or utilizing chemotherapy. This is also known as delaying the "time to cytotoxic chemotherapy."

- Delaying the time before more treatments were needed (also known as "reduction in the risk of starting a new antineoplastic therapy").

- Reducing PSA or controlling PSA and delaying the time before there was an increase in PSA or progression in PSA (also known as "PSA-progression-free survival").

Men with diagnosed mCSPC have options of using Erleada, Xtandi, or Zytiga. However, it should be kept in mind that docetaxel chemotherapy for an average of six cycles over approximately 15 weeks has also been used for mCSPC, in some cases. It is recommended in some men, for example, with "high-volume" mCSPC.

The average treatment time of an ARI or ASI is months to years (continuous use). Docetaxel has minimal out-of-pocket costs, but there are unique side effects including peripheral neuropathy (nerve injury), reduction in neutrophils (type of immune/white blood cell that fights infections), and fatigue, to name a few. (See chemotherapy chapter for more information.) Again, the question is no longer whether these therapies work in mCSPC, but rather which option could be the right one for you.

Non-metastatic castration-resistant prostate cancer (nmCRPC, also known as "M0 CRPC")

Note: All three ARI drugs (Erleada, Nubeqa, Xtandi) are FDA approved and have similar, but also different side effects.

Important treatment note: It is critical to reiterate the remarkable advances occurring in imaging, not just in prostate cancer, but also internal images, that were covered in chapter one (please also refer to the appendix on the latest imaging technology).

PET/CT scans are changing the landscape of nmCRPC by detecting prostate cancer earlier than ever imagined! Some scans can potentially find prostate cancer or pick it up with a PSA of around 0.2. Men with rising PSA numbers could have their cancer located in the body earlier than ever in the history of this disease. These scans can now find cancer in the prostate, the areas around the prostate, nodes, bones, organs, etc., with much greater accuracy earlier in the disease state. This advancement is incredible, but we also wanted you to be aware of it especially in the case of nmCRPC, because it can be argued that fewer men with prostate cancer today will be found to have nmCRPC. Why? The increased use of these amazing scans will find cancer today in someone who otherwise would have been deemed to have nmCRPC just a few years ago. This is being supported right now by ongoing studies of men who would have been considered nmCRPC from using other scanning devices, but now they are finding precisely where the smaller metastatic spots exist, if at all.

Given this background knowledge, it is also important to reiterate that rather than micro-dissecting all the different treatment benefits and clinical trials, the generalized benefits of these approved drugs are summarized in the next paragraph.

All three drugs in their respective individual phase 3 trials enrolled patients with PSA doubling times (DT) of 10 months or less, and all three drugs + ADT prevented metastasis from occurring better than Placebo + ADT. This is also known as an extension or improvement in "metastasis-free survival" (MFS). Keep in mind that a PSADT of 10 months or less usually indicates a more aggressive prostate cancer, so it is exciting that all three drugs helped men in this situation. MFS was improved by each of these drugs and MFS was the "primary endpoint" or the primary goal when these studies were initiated.

In addition, each of these drugs demonstrated some type of additional or "secondary endpoint" or even exploratory endpoint benefits from potentially improving overall survival, delaying PSA progression, delaying pain progression ("time to pain progression"), delaying the time before experiencing some symptoms including delaying the time to a first symptomatic skeletal event (SSE), or delaying the time when chemotherapy would be needed ("time to cytotoxic chemotherapy") or delaying the time to the "initiation of subsequent antineoplastic therapy" (other treatments).

In short, these drugs slow or delay the progression of advanced prostate cancer, and in doing so are potentially able to improve overall survival, or extend life, and delay numerous impacts of advanced prostate cancer. In other words, each of these drugs were incredibly effective at treating some or multiple aspects of nmCRPC (also known as M0 CRPC). Since effectiveness is not the issue, the discussion with your medical team should focus on side effects and issues such as your history and personal preferences. It is easy to get caught in what we term "micro-analysis" where each drug is compared or analyzed based on every single finding, but this is another of the many reasons your medical team is so valuable. They can walk you through the findings or even side effects they consider "clinically valuable" versus "clinically trivial" based on their knowledge and experience, and in working with you personally and understanding your preferences.

(**Note:** None of these medications + ADT were tested head-to-head in nmCRPC, but rather against placebo + ADT, which is another reason we did not want to try and micro-analyze possible treatment differences.)

Metastatic castration-resistant prostate cancer (mCRPC)

Note: Xtandi (enzalutamide), Yonsa (abiraterone), and Zytiga (abiraterone) are all FDA approved for mCRPC

Important treatment note: Again, rather than micro-dissecting all the different treatment benefits and clinical trials, the generalized benefits of these approved drugs are the following:

- Xtandi or Zytiga has demonstrated an overall survival benefit for men with CRPC in phase 3 clinical trials.

- Multiple other potential benefits were observed with the drugs approved for mCRPC including reducing progression of cancer ("radiographic progression-free survival"—also called "rPFS"), extending or prolonging the time needed until chemotherapy was used, delaying the time until first skeletal-related event (SRE), delaying the time needed for opiate drug use for prostate cancer-related pain, delaying the time in ECOG performance status change, delaying the time to functional status decline (helps to maintain quality of life), delaying the time of PSA progression, and more patients had 50% or greater reduction in PSA with treatment.

Common and Not Common Potential Side Effects of the ARIs and ASIs from A-to-Z

The benefits of these medications clearly outweigh the disadvantages for many men, which is the reason these drugs were FDA approved. However, we promised to provide a through overview of common and not-so-common side effects from A-to-Z, which could help in your personal discussions of which pill may be a better fit for you.

Cardiovascular Disease (CVD), or CVD events (arrhythmia, cardiac failure, heart attack, stroke, etc.) risks, and/or the risk of becoming metabolically heart unhealthy can increase with any of these drugs—but how much more?

Cardiovascular disease (CVD) is the leading cause of death in men, as well as in men overall with prostate cancer. CVD also occurs in men with CRPC. Therefore, when most men start any form of localized or advanced prostate cancer treatment they are often already at some increased risk of CVD. Traditional ADT can further increase CVD risk by causing metabolically unhealthy changes such as unhealthy weight or waist gain. There also appears to be little doubt from clinical trials that ARIs and ASIs further increase the risk of cardiovascular disease (CVD), or some markers of an increased risk (some aspect of blood cholesterol—LDL, triglycerides, blood glucose, blood pressure, etc.) or of CVD events themselves (heart attack, stroke, etc.).

What will be argued for some time is the actual amount of risk each drug causes for the individual taking it. This should be discussed with your medical team, particularly if there is a history of established CVD, or a past CVD event. Part of the increased CVD risk could theoretically be reduced by adopting a healthy lifestyle, using preventive medication(s) when needed, and adhering to regular medical visits. Keep in mind, family history or genetics, health access or disparities, previous CVD history (or not) before starting cancer treatment all play a part in your overall risk. Please discuss your current risk of CVD with your healthcare team, how any pill or treatment can change that risk and what you can do about it.

As an example, in the LATITUDE phase 3 Zytiga trial for mCSPC, patients with significant cardiac, adrenal or hepatic dysfunction/issues were not allowed in this trial because of the risk of making their conditions worse. One of the most concerning side effects from this and other phase 3 trials was the higher rate or severity of grade 3-4 hypertension (high blood pressure), which occurred in 20% of the participants in the LATITUDE trial. The point being you must assume all of the drugs in this chapter have the potential to increase CVD risk, CVD events, CVD risk markers, and potentially cause other common and unique issues.

Chemotherapy?

This is not a side effect but a two-tailed side benefit. Many of these prostate cancer pills delay the time needed for chemotherapy. However, there are also some cases of aggressive prostate cancer that could benefit from chemotherapy if given earlier in the advanced prostate cancer process. There is more on this in the chemotherapy chapter, but whether you qualify for chemotherapy earlier instead of these pills, or with any other pills, at any point in the process is up to you and your medical team. We just wanted to make you aware of some of the benefits and limitations of waiting to start chemotherapy.

Constipation or Diarrhea

PW Lifestyle Empowerment Moment

All of the prostate cancer treatment pills in one clinical trial or another reported constipation or diarrhea as a side effect. Regular exercise and consuming daily healthy dietary fiber sources (e.g., fruits, vegetables, beans, lentils, oatmeal with added flax or chia seed powder, some breakfast cereals, etc.) may reduce the risk of constipation if you also increase your intake of water or improve hydration since it helps fiber work more effectively. It also prevents dehydration from occurring with exercise. Exercise stimulates the bowels to keep moving or to essentially keep the train moving so to speak, so it is not running too slow or too late, but right on time (sorry but this is my favorite analogy). Also, please introduce or increase dietary or even supplemental fiber sources (psyllium, etc.) slowly to give your body and gut a chance to get accustomed to this change.

Furthermore, over-the-counter loperamide (also known as Imodium and similar generic brands of anti-diarrhea medication) is one of the most tested and effective products to reduce the duration and potential severity of diarrhea. Please ask your medical team if you should carry or have at home some loperamide if or when diarrhea occurs.

Total daily dosages and pill sizes currently available:

- **Erleada** daily total dosage is 240 mg
- **Nubeqa** daily total dosage is 1200 mg
- **Xtandi** daily total dosage is 160 mg
- **Yonsa** daily total dosage is 500 mg
- **Zytiga** daily total dosage is 1000 mg

Note: *It depends on the company but, in general, you will need two or four pills (capsules, tablets, etc.) to reach the total daily dosage. So, if two pills are only needed then each individual pill size is larger versus the four-pill option from the same company (for example with Xtandi). Still, the actual size of each pill is not just based on the active ingredients but the inactive ingredients (also called "excipients"). In some cases, outside of prostate cancer, inactive ingredients can make up almost 75% of the pill! If you have difficulty swallowing pills or prefer smaller pills, you can ask your medical team which is the smallest or easiest to swallow.*

Drug Interactions can happen

PW Lifestyle Empowerment Moment

All these drugs either have the ability to reduce or increase levels of other drugs in the body, or other drugs have the ability to reduce or increase the level of ARI or ASI drug exposure themselves. There can also be drug interactions with supplements and even foods and drinks. So, please ask your healthcare team about the latest drug interactions. For example, the supplement St. John's Wort can reduce the effective drug level of Nubeqa in the body. Conversely, grapefruit juice has the ability to increase Nubeqa drug levels in the body. Therefore, you could be minimizing the chance of a response from using a supplement such as St. John's Wort or increasing the chances of serious side effects to the drug when drinking grapefruit juice, and neither situation is good. Additionally, the levels of some statin or cholesterol lowering drugs could increase in your body, increasing the risk of side effects, if taken with Nubeqa. These are just a few examples. All the other prostate cancer drugs have potential unique interactions which should be discussed with your healthcare team. In all fairness, in our review of the drug websites, it appeared that Nubeqa made their drug interactions easier to understand for patients compared to the other medications at the time this book was written.

It is also important to remember that some of these pills could increase the risk of abnormal liver enzyme increases or liver injury and damage. This is yet another reason your medical team should review your list of supplements and prescriptions before taking these pills, to make sure a drug reaction could not increase the already heightened risk of liver problems with some of these medications.

Fall/Fracture risk can increase with some of these drugs

Currently, Erleada and Xtandi are the ARI drugs that could increase the risk of falls or fractures. It does not mean the others cannot (abiraterone needs steroid drugs to be taken with it and if used long term could theoretically result in bone loss), but rather at this time these are the drugs that need to mention this risk based on past clinical trial data.

Fatigue

This is a side effect reported by all the ARIs and ASIs. Traditional ADT also causes fatigue. So, please ask your medical team which of these drugs have the lowest current rate of reported fatigue. If your fatigue is interfering with your activities of daily living (ADL) please ask what other options are available to you. Your healthcare team may suggest switching pills or reducing a dosage.

In the ENZAMET trial of Xtandi for mCSPC clinically significant fatigue occurred in 25% of Xtandi participants versus 14% in the other group. What was learned from ENZAMET was that when this pill was added to someone who had already received chemotherapy there were additional side effects, including fatigue (as expected in some cases). It also indicated that fatigue should be discussed with your medical team.

In the Xtandi PREVAIL trial for mCRPC fatigue was one of the most common reasons to stop using the drug, but this only occurred in 1% of the patients so it was still manageable in many other patients. In the PROPSER trial of Xtandi for nmCRPC there was an increased risk of fatigue or weakness (40% vs. 20% with placebo), which was the most common reason for treatment to be stopped, which occurred in approximately 1.6% of the Xtandi-treated patients, which is again low but still noteworthy.

FDA approvals currently

(which allows for updated safety data)

Here we will repeat FDA approvals for each drug because it allows you to regularly check the respective websites of the FDA and drug companies to see if there are any new safety concerns. Also, it may provide an even greater look at overall and specific safety concerns because you are able to see which drugs have been tested more than others in phase 3 clinical trials. For example, Xtandi is approved for all three advanced prostate cancer forms (mCSPC, nmCRPC, and mCRPC). This is not to imply it is the drug for you since it has been the most tested in various forms of prostate cancer, but rather it allows for looking at the different situations and side effects experienced each time the drug was tested. On the other hand, Nubeqa, which is approved for one type of advanced prostate cancer, also needs to be part of the discussion in terms of the latest updated benefit versus risk data since the drug was FDA approved. Another example is Yonsa, which is a more flexible (with or without food) and lower dosage form of abiraterone (Zytiga) but has not received the type of large-scale phase 3 testing that Zytiga originally accomplished. Do any of these observations make a difference to you or your medical team? We have no idea. What makes a difference to you and your medical team is dependent on so many factors. Again, this is where treatment becomes personalized. So, here are the current FDA indications:

- **Erleada** = mCSPC, nmCRPC
- **Nubeqa** = nmCRPC
- **Xtandi** = mCSPC, nmCPSC, mCRPC
- **Yonsa** = mCRPC
- **Zytiga** = mCSPC, mCRPC

Financial Toxicity/Assistance

To say that many of these pills are not low cost is an understatement. Many people need assistance in paying for them. Please talk to your healthcare team and check the official drug website because most of them have a phone number you can call for further financial assistance ideas whether you have insurance or not. Additionally, your medical team and social worker may offer other drug coverage ideas.

Food or No Food Restrictions?

- **Erleada** can be taken with or without food.
- **Nubeqa** must be taken with food.
- **Xtandi** can be taken with or without food.
- **Yonsa** (abiraterone) can be taken with or without food.
- **Zytiga** (abiraterone) must be taken without food.

Note: *The company making Erleada suggests you could also take your pills with four ounces of applesauce if you are having trouble taking them. These interesting, unique, and more specific instructions are on their website in their downloadable patient brochure.*

Hypertension and at home blood pressure (BP) monitoring

PW Lifestyle Empowerment Moment

ARI or ASI pills, in general, can increase your blood pressure. Ask your physician if you need to also monitor your blood pressure from home. It would seem to make a lot of sense to own a low-cost, high quality home blood pressure monitor, for example from Omron or another reputable company. Discuss a regular schedule of monitoring your blood pressure at home, whether it is every week or a few times a month. Then, record your BP numbers and bring this information each time you visit with your regular medical team. Taking your own BP could play an important role in understanding how well your BP is really doing while on these pills, and if more should be done about it. Additionally, less appreciated and utilized are 24-hour ambulatory blood pressure monitors you can obtain from your health care provider if there is ever a situation where your average blood pressure numbers and changes are too difficult to accurately determine at home or at the doctor's office. These devices collect blood pressure numbers every 30-60 minutes during the day and also record at night. Then all this information can be posted on a computer, resulting in some of the most accurate blood pressure readings during the day and at night when asleep.

"Inactive" ingredients in pills to look out for because they could still be "active." For example, how much lactose?

PW Lifestyle Empowerment Moment

We feel it is important to look at the so-called "inactive ingredient" lists for any over the counter or prescription medication. Although they are called "inactive" (or "excipients"), some of them can be "active" because people with an allergy to the compound could theoretically have an allergic reaction to the pill. For example, approximately, 70-75% of the world population is estimated to be lactose intolerant (LI). And some minority groups have higher levels of intolerance. The degree of intolerance falls into categories suggestive of mild, moderate, or even severe LI. The good news is that most of the lactose found in medicinal pills appears to be low, or in the 100s of milligrams, which does not seem to increase the risk of a reaction (bloating, cramping, etc.). However, for individuals with more extreme or severe forms of LI it would be nice to know the exact dosage of lactose in pills you are taking to help decide, with your medical team, whether these pills work for you.

Since our last check of all the official drug websites it appears that "lactose monohydrate" is found in the inactive ingredients for Nubeqa, Yonsa, and Zytiga, so if you and your medical team are concerned about your LI then please check with the company for the latest approximate current dosage of lactose per single pill. Nubeqa is supposed to be taken with food, so it would be important in some cases to know how much lactose it is contributing to your daily allowance if you are sensitive to lactose. Additionally, many people with LI take lactase pills or dairy products such as milk with Lactaid (or other commercial options) containing the enzyme (lactase), which digests the lactose thus causing minimal issues with lactose. Whether this is an option has not been discussed in the medical literature with these drugs to our knowledge, which is why it should be discussed with your medical team, and the company, if needed for your individual situation.

Joint pain (arthralgia) or musculoskeletal pain (learning from breast cancer)

There are effective estrogen reducing pills ("aromatase inhibitors") used in many breast cancer patients that are known to increase the risk of muscle and joint pain. It is interesting that testosterone reducing/blocking pills for men (ARI or ASI) are now also known to increase the risk of joint and muscle pain. Talk to your medical team about over the counter pain relieving gels, creams, or pills you could use for this side effect or whether applying a heating pad to these areas would also be helpful. When examining the latest beneficial research in this area also look toward breast cancer research and share this information with your team. Multiple preliminary clinical studies thus far in breast cancer have found an overall improvement in musculoskeletal pain with exercise (aerobic and resistance). Other studies using acupuncture, targeted heat, physical therapy, and even stress reduction has been associated with improvement. So, could these same interventions help men? Ask your medical team please.

Liver and kidney function

As mentioned earlier, some of these pills may increase the risk of injury to the liver. For example, in the AA-COU-301 and AA-COU-302 trials of Zytiga for mCRPC, and combining results with the overall collective Zytiga data, the most common reason for stopping the drug was due to liver toxicity (hepatoxicity), along with cardiac issues. Another example was the increased risk of rising liver enzymes (a marker called "AST") in the ARAMIS trial with Nubeqa, although only a small percentage were severe cases of toxicity. Whenever someone already has compromised liver and/or kidney function there is usually even more careful attention paid to any pill or procedure being used in or added to treatment. So, if you have a history of liver or kidney problems please talk to your medical team before adding any new pills to your prostate cancer treatment, and this includes anything over the counter, including CBD or other products.

Prednisone long-term side effects (applies to abiraterone)

Blood pressure and/or blood sugar increases, or even bone loss are just three of the known side effects when taking corticosteroid medications such as prednisone or methylprednisolone for short or long periods of time. If your medical team thinks you will be on abiraterone (Zytiga or Yonsa) for a long time, then closer attention should be paid to these and other potential side effects while on prednisone or prednisone-like drugs.

Men with type-2 diabetes who are taking blood sugar lowering medications must also be careful when taking abiraterone because there have been some serious cases of low blood sugar (hypoglycemia) reported (drug-drug interaction). It should also be mentioned that abiraterone (Zytiga or Yonsa) can increase the risk of edema or swelling in your legs or feet so if you are concerned or already prone to this issue please discuss this with your healthcare team.

Rash? Hypothyroidism?

In the TITAN trial of Erleada (28% vs. 9% with placebo) and SPARTAN (25% vs. 6% with placebo) there was an increased risk of rash. Since this appears to be receiving some recent attention, you can talk with your medical team about the latest information. In the TITAN and SPARTAN trials, the rash usually started (if at all) within 2-3 months of treatment and got better or went away within three months of when it started. It was usually treated with an oral antihistamine drug or topical steroid medication (approximately 19% of patients with rash took other steroid medications). So, it was, in general, a temporary rash. When an Erleada dose was interrupted and then reintroduced, 59% of those previous rash patients experienced recurrence of their rash. In the ARAMIS trial of Nubeqa for nmCSPC rash also occurred, but it was less common compared to Erleada.

There was also a slightly higher risk of hypothyroidism reported in the TITAN (4% vs. 1% with placebo) and SPARTAN (8% vs. 2% with placebo) trial as a side effect in the Erleada group, which also appears to receive some attention. It should be kept in mind that it was based on blood levels of TSH, and few patients required actual thyroid hormone treatment for it. Regardless, it should be discussed with your medical team, especially if you have a history of thyroid issues.

Seizures, crossing the blood-brain barrier (BBB), and central nervous system (CNS) effects (mental health issues)

Erleada and Xtandi can cross what is known as the human blood-brain barrier (BBB), which means these drugs could slightly increase the risk of seizures, especially in those with an increased risk of seizures. In the Xtandi AFFIRM (after chemotherapy) trial seizure was the most common side effect which led to stopping the drug (approximately 1% of patients). It is for this and other reasons when the information became available, patients with a history of seizures were not allowed into the SPARTAN (using the drug Erleada) or PROSPER (using the drug Xtandi) phase 3 trials for nmCRPC. However, Nubeqa appears to either not cross the BBB, or have less drug cross the BBB, and thus patients with a history of seizure were allowed into the ARAMIS phase 3 trial for nmCRPC. What does this suggest for other side effects that could impact brain health such as cognition or memory? It is not known right now, so talk to your medical team about the latest information on these side effects.

In addition, the following rare side effects should also be discussed apart from seizure risk when using these drugs: posterior reversible encephalopathy syndrome (PRES-a neurological disorder); hypersensitivity reactions; and falls and fractures. While warnings regarding these potential side effects are listed on the Xtandi website, there is some debate over whether these warnings or increased risks are related to the crossing of BBB. However, we wanted to let you know about them so you can discuss it with your healthcare team.

Weight Loss?

Traditional ADT can cause weight or waist gain in many men and this has been well known for some time. The ARI drugs, however, appeared to cause some weight loss in many of their clinical trials. But why? Is it because these drugs suppressed appetite or increased fatigue, or was it a result of diarrhea or nausea? In other words, was weight loss caused by the drug mechanism and/or the side effects of the drugs? It would be nice to believe these drugs do not promote weight or waist gain, but the greater point we are reiterating from chapter one is that any change in weight, whether a gain or loss, should be reported to your medical team.

Zytiga or Yonsa requires a steroid-type drug to be used with it, for example prednisone (Zytiga) or methylprednisolone (Yonsa), and these steroid drugs are known to potentially increase the risk of weight gain or make it more difficult to lose weight. Perhaps this is part of the reason weight loss was not reported with these ASI drugs. Regardless, the take home point is the same, which is any noticeable change in weight (down or up) should be mentioned to your healthcare team.

Xofigo (radium 223) with Zytiga/Yonsa (abiraterone)
Not recommended outside of clinical trials

This was mentioned in other chapters but in a study known as ERA-223 with mCRPC there was an increased risk of fractures and deaths in men receiving Xofigo + Zytiga compared to the group receiving placebo + Zytiga. This is why the combination is being discouraged until more is learned from this and other relevant studies. Interestingly, it appears the use of bone-protective agents (BPAs) in some participants of this study offered an advantage in reducing the risk of fractures.

Zzzzz—Sleep! Insomnia and restless leg syndrome (RLS)?

PW Lifestyle Empowerment Moment

Interestingly, most of these prostate cancer drugs demonstrated minimal impact on sleep, including insomnia. Why? We have no idea, but it is essential to conclude this section by mentioning that there were not large differences in permanent treatment discontinuation with the drug versus a placebo or comparison group in many of these studies. In other words, despite the long list of potential side effects most participants in these studies tolerated the drug well and more severe side effects were uncommon. Regardless, back to the sleep issue. Is it because of fatigue that some men had no issues sleeping? Was it underreported or treated before the study started? Insomnia or issues with sleep are common underappreciated cancer side effects, as well as side effects of some medications, so please talk to your medical team if you are having any issues with sleep.

For example, a study of Zytiga showed a slight increased risk of insomnia and that could have been due to the use of prednisone with it because it is well-known these steroid type medications can disrupt sleep. However, in two Xtandi trials (ARCHES & PREVAIL) for example, there was an increased risk of restless leg syndrome

(RLS), which is known to disrupt sleep in the person experiencing it and can also impact the person sleeping next to the person experiencing it. Does RLS increase in some of the drugs that cross the blood brain barrier or BBB (see seizure side effect)? Anti-seizure drugs have treated RLS in some cases, but Erleada crosses the BBB and did not seem to cause RLS. Was it due to an iron deficiency in these patients (one of the known treatments for RLS in some cases is iron)? Again, we do not seem to know, but it is remarkable how little we do know about sleep, sleep issues, and many of these prostate cancer treatments (unlike the situation in breast cancer for example). Regardless, there are plenty of options to improve sleep quality and quantity today, from over the counter (OTC) remedies, to lifestyle or behavioral changes (sleep hygiene).

PW Lifestyle Empowerment Moment:

Androgen supplements could be a problem. Potassium-rich foods are usually heart-healthy foods, but do not take Zytiga with food (only Yonsa with food).

Patients should not take any androgen-like hormonal dietary supplements such DHEA, Tongkat ali (Eurycoma longifolia), Tribulus terrestris, or any other potentially testosterone-increasing supplement while taking ASIs (and arguably ARIs), or when dealing with prostate cancer, because these products could potentially reduce the efficacy of these drugs and other treatments. DHEA and other supplements advertised to increase androgens could be turned into testosterone by the body and tumor cells. In other words, since Zytiga also blocks DHEA from being produced, then taking DHEA or other androgen-like products is potentially giving prostate tumors precisely what the drug is trying to prevent them from getting in the first place—more keys to fit into those locks that could result in more growth.

Another concern, which Zytiga and Yonsa (abiraterone) highlight is the side effect of low potassium levels. Individual potassium supplements can be toxic in higher dosages, and if potassium is needed then your medical team can help. However, still being aware of potassium-rich foods, in general, is a good thing for most individuals with and without prostate cancer. Dietary sources of potassium usually contain multiple other healthy ingredients. For example, avocados are high in fiber, potassium, magnesium, healthy fats, with some protein, and almost no cholesterol, sodium, sugar, etc. and they are nutrient-dense (not nutrient-deficient like so many processed or ultra-processed foods). Most fruits and vegetables contain healthy amounts of potassium, and they are also nutrient-dense. Nuts, seeds, chocolate (sorry, but we had to throw that in—everything in moderation) are also good sources of potassium. Please google the top sources of "dietary potassium" and slap the list on the refrigerator so you can get healthy sources of potassium and improve your overall diet. Just remember, people with kidney disease may have to restrict their intake of potassium, but many people have a tough time getting sufficient potassium from foods or meeting those daily adequate intakes because it means eating healthy on a regular basis. Again, talk to your healthcare team about diet and not just supplements.

Please also keep in mind that you should never take Zytiga with any food—only a glass of water. Why? This could make side effects worse, even life-threatening, due to overexposure of some of the ingredients.

Final Important Note

This was the most difficult chapter of the book to write because of the numerous pills available for various situations, and because of the common and not-so-common side effects of each one. This chapter was originally twice as long, but we reduced it by half as we drew closer to the publication date. It just demonstrates, as always, why open communication with your medical team on the benefits and side effects are so crucial. Even after spending hundreds of hours to make this chapter objective and understandable it still does not come close to being as effective as an open discussion with the medical team you entrusted with your treatments. However, if this chapter provides you with just a few extra thoughts or questions to discuss with your medical team that you had not previously known about, then we have done our job. Thank you as always for reading all this information. Keep in mind, with all the different drugs in this chapter there are bound to be changes on a regular basis in terms of efficacy and side effects.

Notes:

_____
_____
_____
_____
_____
_____
_____
_____
_____
_____
_____
_____
_____
_____
_____
_____

CHAPTER 5

Chemotherapy

Taxotere and Jevtana

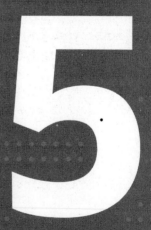

5

PW Quick & Concise Chapter Summary

Chemotherapy is arguably one of the most misunderstood terms within prostate cancer treatment. The perception can be very different from reality because not only does chemotherapy have the proven ability to improve survival or extend life in CRPC patients, but it could also improve quality of life in some patients by helping control or reduce cancer progression. As a result, it could then reduce some of the symptomatic burdens caused by these tumors (pain, etc.). Taxotere (also known as "docetaxel") and Jevtana (also known as "cabazitaxel") are the two FDA approved drugs for metastatic CRPC and both drugs have been shown to prolong life/improve survival. Taxotere is usually the first chemotherapy drug used in CRPC, while Jevtana is usually the second chemotherapy drug used after Taxotere is no longer an option. Both IV chemotherapy drugs are typically given every 3 weeks (it takes about an hour), but the timing and dosage of these drugs has some flexibility based on research, your specific situation, and discussions with your medical team. Daily prednisone pills are also approved for use with these drugs to help reduce the side effects. The daily prednisone or steroid drug needed to control side effects has been a part of all the major clinical trials of these chemotherapy drugs, so they are also an important part of the chemotherapy efficacy and safety process. Both Taxotere and Jevtana are a part of the "Taxane" class of drugs because they were produced from material found in the European Yew Tree (also known as "Taxus baccata"). A phase 3 trial known as TROPIC found Jevtana improved survival in men with CRPC that were no longer able to continue with Taxotere. Another trial known as PROSELICA found there is some flexibility with Jevtana dosing. In addition, a phase-3 trial known as FIRSTANA provided a head-to-head comparison of Taxotere versus Jevtana and found some side effects similar and some that are unique to each chemotherapy drug, which could help in your discussions with your medical team. Chemotherapy has been and continues to be tested in earlier stages and situations against prostate tumors in combination with other drugs and therapies to determine if it could help prevent this disease from returning or progressing. Promising results already exist that should be discussed with your medical team.

Chemotherapy—

Perception differs from reality because of the efficacy, potential quality of life benefits and versatility throughout prostate cancer.

Chemotherapy is a tough word for many people to hear because it can be associated with a long list of negative side effects and toxicity. However, in prostate cancer, as with some other cancers, the reality is that chemotherapy has not only improved the quantity of life of many patients, but also the quality. The quality? Yes, this is one of the most surprising findings for patients—that chemotherapy can reduce some of the tougher symptoms caused by advanced prostate cancer. Chemotherapy is in fact being tested and even used in some select cases today for more aggressive prostate cancer at earlier stages of the disease, combined with other therapies to try and reduce relapses, progression, or metastasis. Some of these tests include the ongoing PEACE-1 phase 3 trial using combinations of Taxotere, Zytiga, ADT, or radiation, which is already demonstrating and reporting some beneficial results, and should be discussed with your medical team, and the ongoing PEACE-2 phase 3 trial looking at the combination of ADT, radiation, and chemotherapy (Jevtana) for more high-risk localized and metastatic hormone sensitive (CSPC) prostate cancer. Other notable published phase 3 trials known as "CHAARTED" or "STAMPEDE" have already found potential benefits when using Taxotere earlier in some high-risk ADT sensitive (CSPC or HSPC-hormone sensitive prostate cancer) men with locally advanced or metastatic prostate cancer.

Most men (approximately 80%) in these clinical trials were able to complete all the intended six cycles of treatment of Taxotere chemotherapy required or needed. Side effects were not the limiting factor in these studies, which were published many years ago, so perhaps limited public knowledge or awareness of these other novel clinical trials and potential uses for chemotherapy could be a limiting factor? There is a perception and then there is the reality.

Again, it is very easy to perceive newer therapies getting approved as better or less toxic compared to chemotherapy, but this is not always true. For example, ADT causes numerous potential side effects and often impacts normal tissue as well as cancer tissue—but this is not labeled or called "chemotherapy." Other newer drugs in this book also increase the risk of diverse side effects while eliminating cancer cells, but again, are not called chemotherapy. In other words, the word chemotherapy has perception that is difficult to "shake off." This perception may always be difficult to minimize, but the beneficial reality is what should receive more attention—similar to the other effective drugs in this book. The real questions to ask are when, where, and how to use these treatments, while preventing and treating side effects. When used at the appropriate time these therapies can result in profound potential benefits. Therefore, the purpose of this chapter is to better see the advantages and disadvantages of these proven treatments and specifically discuss them with your medical team to determine what is right for you.

Taxotere and Jevtana—

could be considered "naturally" derived medicines working to reduce or stop cancer cell growth.

Both Taxotere and Jevtana could be considered naturally derived medicines because they come from parts of the European Yew Tree, which is also known as "Taxus baccata." This is part of the reason their drug class is commonly referred to as the "Taxanes." Of course, they are now primarily manufactured in the laboratory, which not only helps to preserve these unique medicinal tree sources but allows these drugs to help humans all over the world.

Taxotere and Jevtana are believed to work in several ways, such as causing some injured cancer cells to self-destruct, but primarily they are known to target and interfere with cell division so that cancer cannot rapidly reproduce and grow. As such, they affect the most rapidly growing cancer cells. Unfortunately, chemotherapy drugs cannot, in general, tell the difference between the rapidly growing cancer cells and normal cells of the human body. Therefore, rapidly dividing and growing human body cells are the ones most impacted by side effects. For example, hair, nails, gastrointestinal, and bone marrow cells (the source of red and white blood cells, and platelets) grow relatively rapidly, and side effects have a greater chance of occurring in these areas of the body. Yet, each chemotherapy drug impacts some areas of the body more than others, so these drugs have some similar, but also some unique side effect profiles. To better understand these side effects, you should know about FIRSTANA—the phase 3 clinical trial that compared Taxotere to Jevtana. Although both worked well against CRPC, there were similar and different side effects, which we thought should be mentioned upfront.

FIRSTANA Phase 3 trial—

Taxotere vs Jevtana shows side effects are similar, but also different.

Over 1,100 patients were included in this phase 3 trial. The participants were recruited from 159 medical centers around the world and were patients that had not received chemotherapy for prostate cancer before (also known as "chemotherapy naïve"). Participants received either one of two different doses of Jevtana, or the standard dose of Taxotere every three weeks along with daily prednisone. Peripheral neuropathy (nerve damage of hands and/or feet), stomatitis (swelling or inflammation of the mouth or lips,) peripheral edema (swelling usually of feet/ankles), alopecia (hair loss), and nail disorders were more common in the Taxotere group, while low neutrophil (one type of white blood cell that fights infections) counts resulting in fever, diarrhea, and hematuria (blood in the urine) were more common with Jevtana.

When it started, participants in this trial ranged in age from 41 to 90 years old. In fact, approximately 20% were 75 years of age or older. PSA of the participants ranged from nearly undetectable to almost 7000, and close to 90% of these participants had bone metastasis. This is important because it not only demonstrates the diverse range of ages and PSA levels chemotherapy could beneficially impact, but also the importance of understanding similar and unique side effects.

Most men with CRPC can tolerate chemotherapy because most men have good performance status or are still functioning well when receiving it (also known as an ECOG performance score of 0-2—please see prognosis chapter). Still, there are individual considerations. For example, for a man with a past or current history of peripheral neuropathy Jevtana could be a more appropriate choice, or for someone extremely concerned about hair loss. However, if diarrhea or further concerns over reducing neutrophil counts are an issue then perhaps Taxotere or even something else would be a better fit. Again, knowing the similarities and differences in side effects, along with the efficacy of these drugs, is what most medical teams are remarkable at doing, so please discuss it with them.

Taxotere is often tried first, and then Jevtana is usually used when Taxotere is no longer effective, not able to be tolerated, or simply not an option anymore.

It was the result of two phase 3 clinical trials that first found Taxotere significantly improves the chance of living longer for men with CRPC. These trials were published way back in 2004, which shows just how long and effective this chemotherapy drug has been within the setting of metastatic CRPC. Many years later, Jevtana was found to benefit men with metastatic CRPC no longer responding to Taxotere in a phase 3 trial known as "TROPIC." Taxotere was also found to reduce pain and improve quality of life for many patients. Many individuals miss these important points when considering the long list of potential side effects associated with Taxotere. Despite this risk of side effects, most of them were mild-to-moderate (also known as "grade 1 or 2"). More severe side effects are known as "grade 3 or 4," and although they occur less frequently with these drugs, it is important to have the discussion with your medical team regarding what grade side effect concerns them the most, based on your individual situation.

For many patients, the overall benefits exceeded the negatives caused by side effects. Oncologists, for example, usually have a lot of experience with Taxotere (docetaxel) because it has been around for so long and approved to treat many cancer types over the years. Also, most of the costs should be covered by insurance.

While the three-week standard treatment of Taxotere (plus daily prednisone) has a proven survival benefit based on phase 3 trials, it has also been studied at a weekly lower dosage in some patients. Both the standard treatment and lower dosage provided quality of life and pain reduction benefits. If Taxotere cannot be given every three weeks for some reason, then there is flexibility on dosages and schedules for medical teams. Commonly, most patients do well enough to receive it every three weeks.

Age does not appear to impact the survival benefit of Taxotere, but in general the healthier the patient at the time of Taxotere treatment, the greater the chance for benefit. Fatigue is often a more common side effect of these chemotherapy treatments, or what is often known as "cancer-related fatigue" (CRF), but this is also the case with most treatments at this stage of prostate cancer.

PW Lifestyle Empowerment Moment

One of the largest and most comprehensive reviews of treatments for cancer related fatigue (CRF) was published in the prestigious medical journal "JAMA Oncology" (Mustian KM, et al) and included over 110 well-designed or methodologically robust randomized clinical trials and over 11,000 participants. This review found amazing benefits with a "magic pill" (in my opinion) that occurred regardless of age, gender, cancer type, or version of the magic pill used. What was the magic pill? EXERCISE! That is right! All three types of exercise appeared to work equally well (aerobic, resistance, or combined). Exercise was found to be one of the best options for CRF and was recommended to be one of the "first-line treatments for CRF." In addition, psychological interventions, such as cognitive behavioral therapy (CBT), were found to be beneficial for treating CRF and were also recommended to be first-line therapies! Exercise or interventions such as CBT were also found to work significantly better than prescription drug options for CRF! "If exercise was a pill, it would receive an immediate Nobel Prize."—Sorry, but I had to throw one of my favorite quotations in there!

More on the Taxotere and Jevtana process, PSA, PSA flare, and side effects

On average, an infusion of either drug generally takes about one hour. The amount of the actual chemotherapy drug is tailored to your body size. This maximizes the effect of the drug, while attempting to minimize the side effects. Using your height and weight within an accepted standardized equation, your medical team determines your body surface area (BSA) in square meters. Next the team multiplies the suggested drug dose to be given by your BSA. For example, if your body surface area is 1.70 square meters and the dose of Taxotere to be given is 75 mg/m2, then the medical team multiplies 75 x 1.70 to get 127.5 mg. If the BSA is 2.0 square meters, then the medical team multiplies 75 x 2.0 to get 150 mg. Thus, the higher the BSA number measured for a person, the larger the potential dosage of drug given. So, if two people weigh the same, the taller one will have more BSA and will get more of the drug. Likewise, if two people are the same height, the heavier one will have more BSA and get more of the drug. The recommended standard dose of Taxotere is 75/mg2 and that of Jevtana is either 20 mg/m2 or in some cases 25 mg/m2.

It is also important to bring some attention to the concern some patients have over regular needle sticks, especially when receiving IV treatments every three weeks for long periods of time. When it comes to chemotherapy, your medical team may also have the option of putting in place a catheter or "port." These are usually inserted in a larger vein in the upper body and simply stay in place for a long period of time with minimal discomfort. The port is then connected to the infusion material every time you come in to receive either chemotherapy drug, so needle sticks are no longer needed. The port allows many people to carry on with all their daily activities and makes it easier for some patients to receive chemotherapy on a regular basis.

Another term to understand is "PSA flare," which comes up on the internet and other places with these and other drugs. PSA flare should be part of early discussions with your medical team as it relates to how you are responding to Taxotere or Jevtana. It is not unusual (not common, but it happens frequently enough to talk about) in several cancers to see tumor markers of progression, such as PSA, actually begin to increase when the first few cycles of treatment are started. This is due to the release of these markers as cancer cells are eliminated or destroyed, or normal cells are being injured. This may also be an indication that the treatment is working in some men.

Taxotere and Jevtana often cause a decrease in PSA, or a favorable change in PSA kinetics when they are working well, but some studies have suggested a small number of men may see an initial PSA rise of a few points or, in some cases, a lot more. This PSA flare does not appear to affect the treatment duration or the overall effect of the treatment. Troubling as it may seem, 10% or more of patients receiving these treatments may experience an initial flare in PSA. Experts suggest at least 2-3 cycles (6-9 weeks) or more of treatment should commonly be given to determine whether an increase in PSA means that the chemotherapy is not working (disease is progressing), or that the increase is occurring because the drug is beginning to work.

We mentioned some of the side effects of Taxotere treatment from the FIRSTANA trial, but there is a longer list of possible side effects with this drug, from higher-to-lower percentage, as reported from other clinical trials. Please keep in mind that it may be possible to prevent or treat some of these side effects if they do occur in your case.

Taxotere—Potential Side Effects:

- Hair Loss (alopecia)
- Fatigue
- Nausea and/or vomiting
- Low white cell blood count (most often neutrophils)
- Diarrhea
- Nail changes
- Nerve damage ("peripheral neuropathy")
- Inflammation of the mouth ("stomatitis")
- Swelling ("peripheral edema")
- Change in taste
- Shortness of breath
- Eye tearing

Again, most of these side effects were mild to moderate. Some may last a day, while others can persist for months or longer (such as hair loss or fatigue). It is important to keep in mind that not all these side effects, or the severity of them, are due to Taxotere. They may also occur because men are on ADT (have low testosterone levels) and other medications at the same time. For example, a low level of testosterone by itself can result in fatigue.

In terms of Jevtana, many potential side effects are somewhat similar to Taxotere. Jevtana side effects are ranked from some of the most common to less common side effects based on well-known phase 3 clinical trials. These trials include those mentioned earlier (FIRSTANA and TROPIC), as well as PROSELIC that compared two different dosages of Jevtana (20 mg/m2 vs. 25 mg/m2). So, this list is only for general guidance for discussion with your medical team and not specific to your situation. Also, most of these side effects with Jevtana (like Taxotere) were grade 1-2 (mild-to-moderate) and not 3-4, which is more severe. In all fairness, since most men with CRPC receive Jevtana after receiving Taxotere then some of the side effects listed below would be expected since it is common to move quickly from one drug to the other. In this case, side effects are "transferred" from one drug to the other and there could be additional side effects, such as a reduction in blood counts, for example.

Jevtana—Potential Side Effects

- Low white cell blood count (most often "neutrophils" or "neutropenia")
- Low platelets ("thrombocytopenia")
- Diarrhea
- Fatigue
- Weakness or lack of energy ("asthenia")
- Nausea and/or vomiting
- Constipation
- Blood in urine ("hematuria")
- Reduced appetite
- Weight loss
- Cough
- Shortness of breath

Again, many of the side effects of Taxotere are somewhat similar to Jevtana, but some others are different. For better clarification, please talk to your medical team because newer studies are being conducted all the time. For example, there was a study known as CARD where 25/m2 of Jevtana was given with prednisone/prednisolone and G-CSF, which is another drug used to potentially reduce toxicity and enhance efficacy. In this study, grade 3-4 side effects were experienced in less than 5% of the cases, except for white blood cell count and red blood cell count decreases, which are more common. Still, your medical team has medication to help reduce the severity of these issues in some cases.

Jevtana was originally created to reduce the risk of drug resistance observed with Taxotere, and again was approved for treatment after Taxotere ("second line"), when cancer has progressed on Taxotere. Medical teams have become very familiar with the overall and specific benefits and limitations of this drug. Most insurance companies cover the cost of it. If there are any coverage concerns or questions, then please talk to your medical team and visit the official medication website if needed. As mentioned in the first chapter, it is a good idea to visit the official website for any drug in this book to get updated information on results, side effects, and potential insurance or coverage assistance ideas and contacts.

PW Lifestyle Empowerment Moment:

Intermittent Fasting (IF) is interesting, and so are other diets and exercise

Partial, periodic, temporary, or voluntarily controlled "caloric restriction," better known as "intermittent fasting" (IF) right before and/or after the actual day of your chemotherapy infusion is being researched now as an option to reduce side effects and/or boost the efficacy of chemotherapy itself. Preliminary research in other cancers has suggested a potential quality of life and/ or other possible benefits when reducing calories for a day or more before and a day or so after treatment. The total amount and sources of calories reduced depends on the specific study. For example, recent research from the medical journal "Blood Advances" (Orgel E, et al.), found reducing some calories and increasing physical activity could increase the effectiveness of chemotherapy for older children and adolescents with a certain type of leukemia. This study ("IDEAL" trial) was one of the only such prospective studies ever conducted in hematologic cancers. There was an unusually high participation rate in this study, which was attributed to the sense of "EMPOWERMENT" (we capitalized their quotation of course) patients and families felt having this as an option. Of course, this is not prostate cancer research, but a preliminary study from multiple reputable U.S. medical centers (USC, UCLA, Harvard, City of Hope, etc.). It is these kinds of studies that will encourage more prostate cancer researchers to investigate this further, so we can have an answer soon. Regardless, it is interesting how diet and physical activity are usually recommended parts of most cancer treatments.

Additionally, a fasting mimicking diet (FMD) in the recent phase 2 DIRECT trial (de Groot S, et al. Nature Communications) also found the potential for side effect reductions with conventional chemotherapy treatment in women with breast cancer. The FMD, or reduction in calories was conducted for three days before, and on the day of chemotherapy treatment. One of the chemotherapy drugs used in this trial was docetaxel or Taxotere (taxane). Again, these are preliminarily exciting results, which were initiated based on positive laboratory research. Other diets are being tested now in a variety of situations. We are not there yet, but the research is getting very interesting.

Still, intermittent fasting, or any dietary change, is not easy. In addition, these diets are not always healthy based on your individual situation, and in many cases, not proven to work. There are currently numerous protocols or versions being tested in multiple clinical trials with a variety of cancers around the world. So, please talk to your medical team about the latest research. It is a very interesting option, but one that should be personalized between you and your medical team, and beyond the scope of this book (for now, but hopefully not in the near future because so many studies are being initiated and completed).

PW Lifestyle Empowerment Moment:
Hair loss in men needs awareness, too.

What has always been perplexing is the lack of attention paid toward hair loss and prostate cancer treatment.

In breast cancer and other cancers, there have been discussions and deference paid to this issue for some time. In prostate cancer, it is a quiet subject that appears to receive minimal attention. Some men are concerned about hair loss and discussing potential prevention (e.g., the "cooling cap") and treatment ideas should be discussed with your healthcare team if you and your partner find this issue to be a priority. Many men appear to want to discuss it but for some reason, beyond the scope of this book, it just does not receive the attention it deserves. There are instances when lifestyle empowerment is about simple education and awareness, and this is one of those moments. Your concerns should be embraced and not just tolerated, so please talk to your medical team.

PW Lifestyle Empowerment Moment

Earlier, we mentioned a guideline statement issued by the ASCO (American Society of Clinical Oncology), which is one of the most respected organizations on cancer in the world. The recent statement was about not using a specific supplement known as acetyl-L-carnitine (ALC) during chemotherapy, especially with the Taxane drugs such as Taxotere, and we believe this should also apply to Jevtana. It appeared to increase the risk of chemotherapy induced peripheral neuropathy (CIPN) and potentially the duration or severity of this condition. It is always important to know what someone should avoid as much as what someone should take during cancer treatment. And, although the supplement ALC has shown promise for several conditions outside of cancer, there is currently no apparent benefit and some serious potential detriment when using it during some cancer treatments that already increase the risk of CIPN. Perhaps more exciting in this area are clinical trials showing a potential benefit of acupuncture to reduce the severity of CIPN.

In addition, some medical teams will recommend cryotherapy (i.e., some type of temporary slight cooling measure of the hands, feet, or even scalp) during certain chemotherapy treatments to reduce the risk of CIPN, nail disorders, and hair loss. Some temporary cooling of these areas right before, during, and perhaps for a brief time afterward (the best and most effective regimen is still being tested) constricts blood vessels in these areas and appears to reduce the amount of the chemotherapy drug reaching these extremities, which usually do not have cancer in them. Therefore, it is potentially acceptable, with the approval of your medical team first (please), to reduce blood flow temporarily and slightly to these extremities. Some medical teams are suggesting hands and feet be temporarily placed in specially designed "cooling gloves," "cooling socks," or "cold or cooling caps," which can be purchased by the office or online. There are also ongoing studies using covered ice packs for brief periods (too much exposure could cause frostbite effects) on these same body areas. Regardless, ask your healthcare team about preventing and treating CIPN, nail damage or injury, and hair loss with some of these methods, which have been used in breast cancer for some time.

Other "chemotherapy" drugs are getting tested all the time, as well as "non-chemotherapy drugs."

Older and newer chemotherapy drugs are being tested all the time in clinical studies of men with prostate cancer. For example, carboplatin, cisplatin, doxorubicin, alternative forms of paclitaxel, and others are being tested in a variety of situations, along with ongoing studies of Taxotere or Jevtana, as mentioned earlier.

Note: *As we conclude this chapter on chemotherapy, please keep in mind there are commonly accepted dosages and schedules of how much and when to receive any specific chemotherapeutic drug, but some medical teams may slightly alter these dosages and schedules to best fit your current individual needs and situation. This flexibility is yet another benefit of chemotherapy, like most effective prostate cancer drugs.*

Notes:

_____

_____

_____

_____

_____

_____

_____

_____

_____

_____

_____

_____

_____

_____

_____

_____

_____

_____

_____

_____

_____

_____

_____

_____

CHAPTER 6

Radiopharmaceuticals

Xofigo and Radioligand Therapies: Pluvicto

Note: *Lutetium-177, also known as Pluvicto, was approved by the FDA. Patients should be discussing this potential option, along the others in this book with their medical team because it adds to the overall optimism occurring within prostate cancer research.*

PW Quick & Concise Chapter Summary

Xofigo (also known as "alpharadin," "radium-223 dichloride," or "Ra-223") is approved for CRPC patients with symptomatic bone metastasis and no evidence of visceral (organ) cancer. It is given as six intravenous injections. Each one of these injections take about one minute to give and are separated by approximately 4-week treatment intervals, so the entire treatment process is usually completed within six months. Xofigo contains alpha particles, meaning it contains high-energy radiation that selectively binds to areas of high bone turnover, which are usually the primary sites of bone metastasis. Alpha particles also travel shorter distances when they reach their target to provide damage to prostate cancer tumors that have metastasized to the bones, but at the same time reducing the impact on surrounding healthy areas.

This is the first radiopharmaceutical in prostate cancer history to improve overall survival or extend life. It also significantly reduced or delayed the time to a first skeletal-related event (SRE) and increased quality of life. Many patients received some relief from bone pain in a short time after beginning treatment. This and other types of radiation that are delivered at or into the bone can reduce or impact normal blood cell production, as well as platelets needed for clotting. Diarrhea can also occur, but overall, there is a low risk of grade-3 and -4 (more severe) side effects.

Xofigo is often given when a CRPC patient is no longer responding to chemotherapy, or not able to receive chemotherapy. If the cancer is in places other than the bones, for example, the lymph nodes or organs, then this drug does not impact those non-bony cancerous sites. Again, it is for men with CRPC and symptomatic bone metastasis and without visceral metastasis.

In general, it does not cause PSA reductions, and appears to improve survival by other methods, and we know from the chapter on immune therapies that some unique successful drugs work whether or not PSA is reduced. However, in some patients there is the potential for "PSA flare" with Xofigo, or "pseudo-progression" where initially a PSA will increase as cancer cells are destroyed and release their contents, but the cancer is not actually progressing, and you could still be responding to treatment. Whether or not PSA flare is happening to you is something your medical team can easily detect by using other markers such as imaging tests, ALP and LDH blood tests, among others.

Radio-ligand therapy with lutetium-177, also known as Pluvicto, is another type of treatment able to target metastatic sites using an imaging test (PSMA PET/CT) to identify if you have an important marker ("target") generally found on most prostate cancer cells (PSMA), which determines whether you are a good candidate. The phase 3 VISION trial included patients with cancer progressing PSMA-positive metastatic CRPC (mCRPC) receiving lutetium-177 therapy and standard of care (SOC) versus SOC alone, and recently reported an overall survival (OS) benefit. This is the most recent drug approved for CRPC.

Interestingly, this treatment essentially targets and fights cancer cells in different areas of the body that express PSMA, which suggests it can potentially treat multiple areas of the body impacted by prostate cancer including lymph nodes, some organs, bone, prostate, etc. It also appears to make a big difference to watch when and what you eat, drink, or take before numerous PET/CT scans, including PSMA-based scans!

ALSYMPCA—

the Phase 3 trial that helped Xofigo get approved as the first radiopharmaceutical drug to improve overall survival (OS)

A phase 3 trial known as "ALSYMPCA" (Alpharadin in Symptomatic Prostate Cancer Patients) involved over 900 participants and helped Xofigo get FDA approved. During the trial, CRPC patients with symptoms including those with two or more bone metastasis, but no visceral (liver or lung) metastasis, and no lymph nodes larger than 3 cm on an imaging test received Xofigo or a placebo. No participants with organ or a large lymph node cancer were allowed in this study because men with CRPC and large amounts of prostate cancer outside of the bones are less likely to respond to Xofigo that specifically targets the bone. Participants had either no longer adequately responded to Taxotere (docetaxel), or were unfit for chemotherapy, which included ineligibility or refusal to be treated with Taxotere. Almost 60% of the men in this trial had previously received Taxotere.

Many of the participants had very serious or severe CRPC when the trial began, and the primary question this study was trying to answer, and did successfully, was whether Xofigo improved overall survival (OS). In fact, during the interim analysis of the study, the monitoring committee recommended stopping the study because there was clear evidence of an overall survival benefit favoring Xofigo. Other clinical endpoints of the study also favored Xofigo. For example, the time to the first skeletal-related event (SRE) was longer or delayed in the Xofigo group. Overall, side effects were similar to the placebo in this study except for diarrhea that occurred in 25% of the men receiving the drug versus the placebo, but grade-3 or -4 (more severe) diarrhea was found in only 2% of both groups. Approximately 13% of the participants in the Xofigo group had to discontinue the study because of side effects compared to 20% on the placebo. Grade-3 or -4 lower white blood cell counts or neutropenia (a type of white blood cell that fights infections) were 2% with Xofigo and 1% in the placebo group. And grade-3 or -4 thrombocytopenia (low platelet count) was 6% with Xofigo and 2% with placebo.

The FDA approval of this radiopharmaceutical represented an amazing advancement in this area of prostate cancer research. In the past, other radiopharmaceuticals have been used on men with CRPC primarily for "palliative" use or to try and reduce symptoms, such as bone pain and other skeletal complications of bone metastases. While other radiopharmaceuticals, such as samarium-153 and strontium-89 were used, none had demonstrated a survival benefit until Xofigo was tested and approved.

More on Xofigo—

a calcium copycat and magnet, PSA, and PSA flare (pseudo-progression)

Xofigo acts as a "calcium mimic" or copycat that naturally gets into new bone growth or metabolism in and around the metastatic bone site. This happens because, like calcium, it is also drawn into areas of high bone turnover, which usually results from metastatic bone sites. Therefore, using this drug makes sense against bone metastasis in some men, especially when it can emit radiation at the site of the metastasis itself.

Xofigo contains high-energy alpha particles within a short distance of less than 10 tiny cell diameters. As a result, the bone tumors are more impacted compared to the surrounding healthier areas around the metastatic site. Past radiopharmaceuticals (beta-emitting particles—samarium or strontium) were smaller in size, did not appear to provide this same specific benefit, and did not appear to deliver as much maximum energy to the tumor itself. As mentioned in the chapter on bone-protective agents (BPA), some prostate cancer cells in the bone become chaotic and disorganized, building cells within the bone itself. These cells try to build or make bone, but they are not good at doing it. As a result, they draw or attract large amounts of calcium and phosphate toward themselves and their nearby surroundings. Therefore, one primary pathway whereby Xofigo takes advantage of the cancer is by using its magnetizing action, so to speak, for calcium, getting drawn into and around the area where the cancer is very active. Then, when the drug reaches the cancer target it delivers or releases radiation at the tumor(s) in the bone.

About half the drug is gone after 11 days, so it does not stay in the body too short or long. This is a good thing, because too short could reduce its effectiveness in doing damage to cancer cells, and too long could increase toxicity to the human body (more side effects). After the drug completes its task, it is finally eliminated from the body by the intestines and ultimately excreted in the feces, which is one reason, arguably, why diarrhea was a greater side effect compared to placebo in studies.

What about PSA? In the Provenge chapter on immune therapy we talked about this specific IV drug being effective, despite not usually causing a decrease in PSA—it was helping in other ways yet to be fully discovered. This is essentially the case with Xofigo. A smaller percentage of men experience PSA reductions, but the drug still improves survival in many men (PSA reductions or not). It also reduced some of the symptoms of metastatic CRPC. Medical teams follow many additional prognostic indicators on Xofigo mentioned in the beginning of this book, including imaging tests and other blood tests such as alkaline phosphatase (ALP), lactate dehydrogenase (LDH), and other bone formation or resorption markers which could provide more information in terms of the magnitude of the response, or lack of response, along with other tests your specific medical team is following. Still, medical research teams are always in search of better biomarkers to determine the very best and not so great candidates for these somewhat PSA independent survival therapies, including markers of the degree of response to these drugs. Talk to healthcare your team about how they will monitor your response to this or any other treatment.

In addition, "PSA flare" was discussed in the chemotherapy chapter, where in some cases an apparent initial rise in PSA when starting these drugs, could result in what is known as "pseudo-progression." In other words, the increase in PSA or tracer uptake from the bone scan or another imaging test is temporary and could be partially explained by cancer cells being injured or destroyed, and releasing contents of their cell, including PSA, into the bloodstream. Thus, some of these flares indicate that the drug is beginning to work or working in some men, and in others it could represent real progression based on additional testing. Medical teams today are very good at recognizing and determining within the first few rounds of treatment whether the PSA flare is real or not, and if the drug should be continued.

Other concerns about Xofigo treatment need to be mentioned and even reiterated. Side effects of Xofigo could potentially include the following: nausea, diarrhea, vomiting, and/or peripheral edema (swelling). Also, lower blood cell counts are associated with Xofigo treatment in some patients including the following: low red, and certain immune or white blood cells, such as lymphocytes and neutrophils, as well as platelets. It is also important to mention evidence from a clinical trial known as "ERA-223" which has suggested that Xofigo should not be combined with the drug Zytiga (abiraterone) and prednisone/prednisolone because it may have additive and significant toxicity including an increased risk of fractures and reduced survival. Preliminary information has suggested some men receiving Xofigo should consider being on a bone-protective agent (BPA) for added protection, but again this is preliminary. More evidence on this issue is being collected, so please talk to your medical team about the latest information.

Additionally, preliminary data (not definitive) suggest more than six treatments or higher dosages of Xofigo have not been found to be better than the standard approved total of six treatments, but this continues to be researched at this time.

PW Lifestyle Empowerment Moment

The company that makes Xofigo recognizes something very interesting in their prescription information concerning intestinal movement or elimination of the drug itself from the body. Since the rate at which Xofigo is eliminated from the gastrointestinal tract or feces appears to be impacted by intestinal transit/ movement rates then individuals whose intestines work faster (higher rate) would be expected to eliminate the drug faster, and those with slower rates of intestinal movement would arguably receive more drug to the intestines and theoretically higher intestinal exposure or a higher rate of side effects. The true impact of intestinal movement rates on Xofigo gastrointestinal side effects, such as diarrhea risk or severity was not studied, and this is also acknowledged in the prescription information. However, besides being an interesting future research study, it would appear, at least theoretically, that any lifestyle changes that could accelerate intestinal movement could be potentially helpful.

For instance, aerobic exercise and dietary fiber can both increase gastrointestinal motility. Both are also heart healthy. In other words, even if exercise and dietary fiber are not ultimately found to reduce the side effects of Xofigo, they are still good for your health. Also, it would feel inappropriate to forget about coffee—actually caffeine, which is also known to stimulate intestinal movement. Adding more coffee to this already theoretical side effect reduction plan could also be slightly encouraged, so why not just encourage it anyway? The only caveat to this advice is that there was a higher rate of "dehydration" with Xofigo reported compared to the placebo, so encouraging hydration, or knowing "clear is cool" (from the Provenge chapter lifestyle empowerment moment) is important. Since coffee or caffeine can be considered dehydrating (although this is controversial in moderation), or could encourage dehydration in some patients, it would be wise to drink water before or after your coffee. It should also be emphasized that some of the side effects of Xofigo, for example, diarrhea, nausea, or even vomiting increase the risk of dehydration further, so perhaps the take home message is hydration is important with Xofigo, but so are other lifestyle tips, which also serves a bonus of ultimately increasing your hydration status. For example, most healthy foods have a higher water content, especially vegetables and fruits. In fact, 20-25% of your daily water intake comes from food (not beverages or water itself), so when you consume more dietary fiber, or increase your amount of exercise you should also naturally consume more water. Wow! Lifestyle changes to the rescue once again!

Lutetium-177/Pluvicto—

and a recent successful phase 3 known as VISION, which suggests this will be the next treatment widely available.

A new targeted drug treatment ("radioligand therapy") demonstrated successful results in the phase 3 "VISION" trial. This treatment was able to meet both of its primary endpoints or goals in this study, which was significantly improving overall survival (OS) and radiographic progression-free survival (rPFS) in patients with PSMA-positive metastatic CRPC! As a result, this treatment known as lutetium-177/Pluvicto was the latest treatment approved by the FDA for men with CRPC. This is good news as it adds to the many options now available for CRPC patients. Please talk to your healthcare team about this new treatment option. The following paragraphs provide some basic background on this treatment.

There is another interesting word becoming more common in prostate cancer treatment, which is known as "theranostics." The idea here is to combine treatment or therapy with diagnostics, hence the name "theranostics." For example, a well-known molecular biomarker found on many cancer cells is PSMA (prostate-specific membrane antigen), and if your cancer is demonstrated to be PSMA-positive then you could receive a specific treatment that when given seeks out that specific target using a radionuclide product that is like a heat seeking weapon (Lutetium-177) looking for its specific target (PSMA) on cancer cells. Previously, we talked about Xofigo being drawn to areas of high bone turnover, but this new potential therapy would be attracted to cancer cells already positive for PSMA from a specialized PSMA PET/CT scan. The drug or radioactive particle (therapeutic radioisotope) is known as Lutetium-177, and a somewhat similar version of it has already been approved for use in a different tumor type known as "gastroenteropancreatic neuroendocrine tumors (GEP-NETs)"— also known by the commercial treatment name "LUTATHERA" (lutetium Lu 177 dotatate).

So, it appears the future of theranostics has also arrived in prostate cancer treatment! In the phase 3 "VISION" clinical trial mentioned earlier, patients with metastatic CRPC who were also found to have cancer cells positive for the marker PSMA using a PSMA PET/CT scan, either received Lutetium-177 (actually more officially known as "Lu-177-PSMA-617") with best standard of care (SOC), or best SOC alone. The drug was given once every six weeks, with a maximum of six total treatments. Patients in this trial had to have a castrate level of testosterone (<50 ng/dL or <1.7 nmol/L), one or more metastatic lesions, already received at least one of the newer ARI or ASI (novel anti-androgen axis drugs or medications such as Xtandi, Zytiga, etc.) oral drugs and previously treated with at least one, but no more than two taxane chemotherapy drugs. This new therapy also appears to lower PSA in many patients as it fights prostate cancer. We are eagerly waiting for more information on other potential results such as reductions (or not) in pain because asymptomatic and symptomatic patients were in the VISION trial, quality of life, and more. Patients in this trial had also not recently received another radiopharmaceutical drug. We are also eager to see what documented side effects occurred during this phase 3 clinical trial, and in what percentage of patients along with the number of grade-1 and 2 (less severe) versus grade-3 and -4 (more severe) side effects.

Another potentially very exciting observation with this new drug needs to be mentioned. Lutetium-177/ Pluvicto, again, is directed toward PSMA expression on prostate cancer cells, so it could also target or treat cancer in multiple locations in the body such as the lymph nodes, bones, some organs, prostate, etc., unlike Xofigo, because Xofigo targets prostate cancer metastasized to the bones. So, there are a several settings where this radioligand therapy is being tested including before and after other CRPC treatments, with PARP inhibitors, or immune therapies, to name a few. So please ask your medical team if and where this might fit in your clinical trial, current, or future treatment situation.

Lutetium-177 is a beta-particle, and beta-particles are essentially electrons, which are very small. As mentioned earlier, it was originally thought that this smaller size would be limiting and could cause collateral damage to healthy tissue—not just cancer cells. However, since Lutetium-177 moves toward a PSMA target then the smaller size in this situation could also be advantageous by not only damaging PSMA expressed cancer, but also potentially non-PSMA expressed prostate cancer next to where the damage occurs. In other words, it could (hopefully) cause damage to cancer cells and collateral damage to other non-PSMA expressed adjacent cancer cells. Many prostate cancer cells have PSMA, but some do not—there is a heterogenous mix in many cancers.

Regardless, it would also suggest that Lutetium-177 carries some common and unique side effects. Therefore, it is also critical to discuss the specific possible side effects from this newer potential treatment from other past studies. Reported side effects included dry mouth ("xerostomia"—temporary or permanent), nausea, fatigue, overall and specific blood cell changes (e.g., platelet reductions, etc.). Whether these side effects are more mild-to-moderate or manageable (grade 1-2), or more severe (grade 3-4), will be better known as more information becomes available. Please ask your medical team about what is currently known in regarding common and uncommon side effects of this therapy because this is as important as the efficacy of any treatment.

Numerous other radioligand compounds (e.g., Actinium-225, etc.) are also being studied right now, which makes this new area of treatment very exciting!

PW Lifestyle Empowerment Moment

Diet and supplements have the potential to play an unusually important and even concerning temporary role in the future of PET/CT scans, such as PSMA, which is used with the radioligand treatment Lutetium-177/ Pluvicto mentioned earlier. This issue was also discussed earlier in chapter one under educational tip number 15, but it is worth briefly reiterating and elaborating further here because it is so relevant to the topic of current and future scans and their use in radioligand therapies. When and what you eat or do within a day or more of some scans could impact the reading or accuracy of the results. Choline PET/CT recommends patients should fast (without food or drink) at least six hours before the scan, while Axumin PET/CT instructions recommend fasting for at least four hours before the scan and to avoid "significant" exercise 24 hours before the test.

Now, with that as a fascinating reminder and background let us get back to lutetium-177. It uses a PET/CT PSMA type compound that can be picked up, attached, or ingested by cancer cells and then the scan lights up where the PSMA made contact. Then, if you are a good candidate, lutetium-177 is given and seeks out those targets. When it reaches them, it releases energy and causes damage to the cancer. What is not easy to appreciate is that PSMA stands for "prostate-specific membrane antigen," but like PSA it is not always prostate specific. In addition, although it is found on most prostate cancer cells it can also be found in other types of cells or tissues. It is for this reason Lutetium-177 and other similar compounds have "dry mouth" as a potential side effect because there are areas in the mouth, such as the salivary glands that take up Lutetium-177. Energy is also released in this location causing damage to the saliva making machinery of the body. But the lifestyle story gets more interesting.

Facial ice packs have been used with some success to reduce the uptake of this compound to the salivary glands (even Botox injections are being tested in some studies). But what if you could simply just block the uptake of Lutetium-177 in the salivary glands with a food molecule, and eliminate or reduce this side effect? In theory, this was a really good idea. And, at the time this book was being published several groups, from UCLA to the University of British Columbia, have tried in preliminary studies to accomplish this with a well-known compound found in some foods. What was the common dietary compound they were trying to use? MSG! Also known as "monosodium glutamate"—the food ingredient and additive. I am not kidding here. It made sense to try this because another name for PSMA is "glutamate carboxypeptidase II," which means the compound or amino acid "glutamate" is common to both PSMA and MSG.

However, even though this approach appeared to initially work it simultaneously compromised the tumor uptake of the PSMA compound used to detect the actual tumors. The ingested MSG circulated to other cancerous spots and appeared to block the ability of the PSMA PET/CT to fully light up in the areas that contained cancer. The take home point is now clear but needs far more attention: Whenever you get any type of PET/CT scan using any molecule to try and light up the cancer, please make sure you know the latest lifestyle or dietary instructions regarding what you should avoid and for how long before the scan is done! This is critical because I believe this is one of the most underappreciated impacts of diet and exercise before crucial PET/CT and other scans.

Whether it is MSG, choline, glucose or other compounds that are a ubiquitous part of the human diet there is so much more that needs to be learned on what impacts the accuracy of imaging tests. MSG, for example, is found in so many food products that this needs even more attention. It can be found in fast foods, chips/snack foods, low-sodium seasoning blends, frozen meals, processed meats, soups, sauces, dressings, condiments, and more. Besides diet, what is the impact of strenuous and/or long durations of exercise within a day or so of these scans? Could it also temporarily interfere with the reading because it may shift metabolism to other areas of the body? This appears to be the case with some PET/CT scans (e.g., Axumin as mentioned earlier). Still, research is looking at all these questions right now, which is why by the time you read this patient lifestyle instructions could further change to enhance the accuracy of the results.

However, what again (this was also mentioned in chapter one under educational message number 15) appears to be currently overlooked, in general, in this entire debate are all the dietary supplements and countless other products that contain glutamine or glutamate (they can be potentially converted into each other). In fact, today there are numerous over the counter products, and even prescription medicines, that contain large amounts of these substances. What about those? Shouldn't they also be temporarily (not permanently) restricted for some time right before one of these scans is performed? I believe it needs to be considered based on the latest data, but at the very least this issue needs to be discussed. So, again, please ask your medical team about the very latest and greatest research in this area of diet, supplements, or other pills and lifestyle changes (exercise, etc.). "Lifestyle changes can change so many aspects of life!" I apologize, but I had to repeat another one of my favorite quotations.

There is no better way to end this chapter than reiterating that what you do, and what you learn, can make a big difference. So, please ask your medical team about the most up-to-date diet and other lifestyle restrictions before you get your next PET/CT or another imaging test. In fact, at the time of this writing some of the top sites for PET/CT PSMA scans are already mentioning not to eat or drink anything, except water, for four, six, or even more hours before the exam. There are also medical sites concerned about excessive exercise at least 24 hours before your scan that could cause false positive results in some areas of the body. This is a great start, but this is such a fascinating and fast-moving lifestyle research subject, which also needs your attention and awareness for better results.

CHAPTER 7

PARP Inhibitors

Olaparib (Lynparza) or Rucaparib (Rubraca) and Other
Unique Biomarker Treatment Qualifying Situations

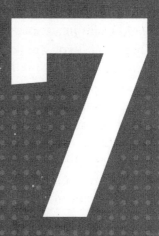

PW Quick & Concise Chapter Review

Studies have now remarkably demonstrated approximately 20-30% of men with metastatic prostate cancer have some type of genetic mutation or alteration that have an impact on cellular DNA repair mechanisms! Again, 20-30%! Therefore, it must also be quite common in many men with any form of CRPC. This means every patient should have a discussion with their medical team about the latest research on unique biomarker testing to determine if they are a candidate for other FDA approved drugs. For example, in the Provenge chapter there was a review of MSI-H (microsatellite instability-high) and other biomarker testing to qualify for an immune drug known as Keytuda (pembrolizumab), as well as other options.

There are two general types of tests that could qualify you for what is known as PARP inhibitor drugs. The first is "germline" testing, which looks at your "inherited" genes from a blood sample (or even buccal or inner cheek swab). The second is "somatic" testing, which examines your cancer tissue or genetic material released into the blood from your cancer to see if they have "acquired" any of these gene mutations that could qualify you for a PARP inhibitor. These drugs are now being used in some types of breast, ovarian, and pancreatic tumors, and are even now available for some CRPC prostate cancer patients. Many patients with CSPC are also being tested for certain biomarkers.

PARPs are a group of enzymes involved in the regular repair of DNA, but a mutation in one of the genes such as BRCA-1, BRCA-2 could result in a cancer unable to adequately repair itself to survive. Therefore, if you are positive for one or more of these biomarker tests then a PARP inhibitor (or another drug mentioned in the Provenge chapter) could be used to exploit this vulnerability in some of your cancer cells. PARP inhibitors take advantage of the fact that some cells are already not able to repair themselves very well when injured. Then the drug further blocks these enzymes to increase the chances that more cancer cells will not be able to repair their DNA, become even more fragile, or even be eliminated. Currently, there are two PARP inhibitors potentially available to

CRPC patients based on germline or somatic testing—"olaparib" (also known as "Lynparza"), or "rucaparib" (also known as "Rubraca")—and potentially several others will be arriving in the near future. Olaparib had a phase 3 trial known as "PROfound," which helped it get FDA approved for a number of mutations including BRCA, and rucaparib had a phase 2 trial known as "TRITON2," which helped it get an accelerated approval for a smaller number of potential mutations including BRCA.

Men with BRCA-2 mutations were the most likely to respond to these drugs from their respective clinical trials. There is a list of common and not so common side effects that should be reviewed with your medical team if you qualify. These unique situations/biomarker testing to qualify for a PARP inhibitor represents a promising and very exciting avenue to potentially receive treatments that were never available to patients! So, the question to ask your medical team is whether you currently qualify for any "germline" or "somatic" cell testing to see if you qualify for other potential prostate cancer or CRPC drugs, such as PARP inhibitors, immune therapies, and others.

PARP—

biomarker testing to qualify for other drugs using germline (non-cancerous cells you were born with or "inherited" mutations) or somatic cells (from your cancer "acquired" mutations) sources, and some PARP Inhibitors are available now!

PARP is the abbreviation for "poly (ADP-ribose) polymerase," which are a group of repair enzymes (proteins) found in normal and cancer cells used for DNA repair. Non-cancerous cells need these repair enzymes so that day-to-day cellular activities can function normally, because cell damage, or errors in cell or DNA replication, happen all the time. If cells were not allowed to repair themselves with this on-site group of "fix-it now" workers, then many diseases could occur at even higher rates than they do now, and even earlier in life. Again, PARP and other repair teams are there to help correct those errors in DNA (genetic material) before they become big problems.

For example, just the day-to-day work or replication of DNA can cause errors. Additionally, daily environmental or lifestyle factors from ultraviolet light (UV) or even background radiation exposure, pollution, tobacco, excessive alcohol intake, and more can cause cellular damage. While PARP works 24 hours a day, 7 days a week to help with DNA repair, cancer cells also rely heavily on PARP in some cases to repair themselves and survive. PARP inhibitor drugs can stop this enzyme from helping cancer cells repair themselves, so they can be eliminated. A cancer cell that is unable to thoroughly repair itself from injury or damage is extremely vulnerable with a serious Achilles' heel that could be exploited by using these PARP inhibitor drugs. The drug is simply taking advantage of their partial vulnerability and increasing the probability the cancer cell becomes even more susceptible or exposed to damage. It is akin to taking a partial hidden defect and turning it into a fully exposed weakness, increasing the odds the cancer cells cannot survive or thrive.

There are two general types of biomarker testing for potential PARP defects and drug qualifications, and both could be available to you right now based on a discussion with your medical team. The first is "germline" testing, where a sample of your "inherited"/non-cancerous cellular material is tested (blood or cheek swab sample) to see if you have any cellular mutations that could put you at a higher risk for certain cancers, or less ability to fight these cancers. The second type is "somatic" testing, which looks at your cancer cells, or a portion of them in the blood or tissue sample that shows whether or not your cancer has "acquired" some mutations over time. Then a drug could be used to exploit those mutations to get a better targeted treatment. So, the question to ask your team is whether you are currently a good candidate for any "germline" or "somatic" cell testing to see if you qualify for other potential CRPC drugs.

This entire field of emerging therapies is part of a growing area known as "precision cancer treatment," or "molecularly targeted treatment." It is one of the newest and most exciting areas of prostate cancer research. While new to prostate cancer, it has been used before and currently in other areas of medicine, such as ovarian cancer treatment with the approval of drugs targeting the BRCA-1 and BRCA-2 gene mutations. BRCA-1 and -2 were thought to primarily place individuals at a higher risk of breast cancer (BRCA = Breast Cancer) or ovarian cancer, but researchers have learned over time that this could also put males at a higher risk of prostate cancer. Also, some prostate cancers, especially as they become more advanced, appear to "acquire" these same and other potential mutations, which can again be exploited by using a drug that targets them.

Studies have now remarkably demonstrated approximately 20-30% of men with metastatic prostate cancer have some type of genetic mutation or alteration that has an impact on cellular DNA repair mechanisms! Again, 20-30%! Therefore, it must also be quite common in many men with any form of CRPC. Many patients with CSPC are also being tested for certain biomarkers.

To reiterate, when these mutations are targeted then DNA damage and some cancer cell destruction can occur.

Currently, PARP inhibitors drugs are an important part of cancer treatment, including some types of breast, ovarian, and even pancreatic cancer. Now, even prostate cancer patients have access to these drugs if they qualify. Soon, other cancers will probably have access to these drugs, and how to best use these drugs, with or without other prostate cancer treatments, will be better understood. There have also been some interesting results from laboratory studies suggesting responses in mutations other than BRCA. This means that many other genetically unstable situations or mutations may quality for some of these medications either now or in the near future.

Before leaving this section, you may be wondering what the impact of PARP is on "normal" human cells with mutations, or could they also block the ability of human non-cancerous cells (not just cancerous ones) to repair DNA? As mentioned, in some cases humans have PARP defects, which not only puts them at increased risk of cancer, but potentially more aggressive cancers.

PARP inhibitors appear to be far more effective or selective, and better able to exploit defects in cancerous cells compared to non-cancerous cells based on past testing. However, some related or unrelated damage in non-cancerous human cells occurs because of the side effect profile of these drugs, which are covered in this chapter.

There are currently two FDA approved PARP inhibitor drugs for certain forms of prostate cancer treatment, known as "Olaparib" (Lynparza) and Rucaparib (Rubraca), and there are others being tested right now!

Olaparib (also known as "Lynparza")—

PROfound phase 3 trial helps it get approved, and the best biomarker candidates for qualifying right now

Here are some important points to consider when discussing olaparib with your medical team:

- The Phase 3 PROfound trial helped this drug get FDA approved in mCRPC patients with BRCA-1, BRCA-2 and ATM gene mutations that failed second generation anti-androgens (ARI or ASI), such as Xtandi or Zytiga. Almost two-thirds of the patients in this trial had received a previous taxane chemotherapy drug, 40% received Xtandi, 38% had received Zytiga, and 20% had received both Xtandi and Zytiga. The median age was 69 years and the age range in this study was age 47 to 91 years.

- Olaparib is an oral drug/pill (generally recommended dosage is 300 mg twice daily, but this can be adjusted based on many factors), which can be taken with or without food.

- Olaparib is officially used for the treatment of adult patients with deleterious or suspected deleterious germline or somatic homologous recombination repair (HRR) gene-mutated metastatic CRPC who have progressed following previous treatment with Xtandi (enzalutamide) or Zytiga (abiraterone). This is a lot of medical vernaculars for saying that ideally patients with metastatic CRPC with DNA damaged repair (DDR) pathways, as demonstrated by germline or somatic biomarker testing, are potential candidates for this drug, especially if they are no longer responding to drugs such as Xtandi or Zytiga. The drug appeared to shrink tumors, slow the progression of the cancer, and improve overall survival in the PROfound trial.

- Some of the mutated mCRPC biomarkers that could potentially qualify a patient include ATM, BRCA-1, BRCA-2, BARD1, BRIP1, CDK12, CHEK1, CHEK2, FANCL, PALB2, RAD51B, RAD51C, RAD51D, RAD54L, etc. This list could change at any moment, and could get larger, or shorter based on the latest research. The two markers that receive the most attention and are often more common are BRCA-1 and BRCA-2. Also, germline testing of BRCA-21 and BRCA-2 would also potentially qualify you for this drug. Interestingly, the largest benefit in the PROfound trial appeared in men with BRCA-2 mutations, which were approximately one-third of the PROfound trial participants.

- Some of the common side effects were anemia (reduction in hemoglobin) and a reduction in other blood or immune cells, fatigue including tiredness or weakness, nausea, reduced appetite, diarrhea, vomiting, cough, and difficulty breathing. Blood clots occurred in more men with olaparib versus men receiving Xtandi or Zytiga.

- It is also important to report that there have been some cases of myelodysplastic syndrome/acute myeloid leukemia (MDS/AML) associated with olaparib (Lynparza), and in some cases they were life-threatening or fatal. Your medical team will monitor you for any signs of bone marrow or blood cell toxicity.

PW Lifestyle Empowerment Moment

You can take olaparib (Lynparza) with or without food, but you also need to AVOID grapefruit, grapefruit juice, Seville oranges and Seville orange juice during treatment with this drug because it could increase the concentration of olaparib (Lynparza) in your blood to an unhealthy level, causing serious toxicity or more severe side effects. It is also interesting that this drug has a warning to be careful when using it with other drugs that could block the metabolism or natural elimination of it via a specific pathway (known as "CYP3A4 inhibitors"). However, cannabidiol or CBD (over the counter and prescription) has been shown preliminarily in some studies to be a strong potential CYP3A4 inhibitor. So, should there also be an immediate warning not to combine this PARP drug with CBD? We do not know, because at the time this book was published we were not made aware of any strong published studies testing this potential drug-drug interaction of olaparib (Lynparza) with CBD from over the counter (OTC) or prescription sources. Please talk to your medical team about the latest information on this potential drug-drug interaction.

In addition, a high fat and high calorie meal can slow the rate of absorption of olaparib by 2.5 hours, but not the eventual extent or amount of the drug absorbed. This suggests if you take these pills with a high-fat meal it could (emphasis on could) take a few extra hours before it is effective. It should still be just as effective when taking it with no food, or with a low-fat meal for example versus a high-fat meal.

Rucaparib (also known as "Rubraca")—

TRITON2 phase 2 clinical trial helped with the accelerated approval and in deciding the best biomarker candidates to qualify for the drug.

Here are some important points to consider when discussing rucaparib with your medical team:

- A phase 2 clinical trial known as "TRITON2," which included over 200 patients with documented DNA repair issues also known as homologous recombination deficiencies (HRD)-positive mCRPC, including 115 with BRCA-mutated CRPC helped allow for the unique accelerated approval of this drug for some CRPC patients. Median age was 73 years and age range in this study was age 52 to 88 years. Patients had received at least one previous androgen-directed therapy and a previous taxane chemotherapy drug. All these patients had a deleterious germline or somatic BRCA mutation.

- TRITON2 was a phase 2 trial versus a more definitive phase 3 trial, so the FDA accelerated approval was based on a suggested potential benefit. Ideally a phase 3 trial would have been better for more definitive benefits and limitations of this drug. Regardless, this is another great potential option, but qualifying is a little more difficult.

- This is also an oral drug (tablet) and the recommended dosage is 600 mg (two 300 mg pills) twice daily for a total daily dosage of 1200 mg with or without food.

- It is officially used for the treatment of adult patients with a deleterious germline or somatic BRCA mutation in metastatic CRPC who have been treated with androgen receptor-targeted therapy and a taxane-based chemotherapy drug. In other words, it inhibits PARP-1, PARP-2, and PARP-3, which again all have some role in DNA repair. In other words, ideally patients with mutations in BRCA-1 or BRCA-2, and only for a cancer that has progressed despite using an earlier treatment with an androgen receptor targeted therapy as well as a chemotherapeutic drug would be the best candidates. Interestingly, like the PROfound trial, patients in TRITON2 were the most likely to respond to the rucaparib PARP inhibitor drug if they had BRCA-2 mutations.

- Some of the common side effects were fatigue such as tiredness or weakness, nausea, anemia (reduction in hemoglobin), liver enzyme test increases (potential liver injury), reduced appetite, rash, constipation, low blood cell counts or low platelets (thrombocytopenia), vomiting, and diarrhea.

- It is also important to report that there have been some cases of myelodysplastic syndrome/acute myeloid leukemia (MDS/AML) associated with rucaparib (Rubraca), and in some cases they were life-threatening or fatal. Your medical team will monitor you for any signs of bone marrow or blood cell toxicity.

PW Lifestyle Empowerment Moment

You can take rucaparib with or without food, BUT a high-fat meal could increase the amount of drug in the blood and delay absorption versus fasting conditions. Caffeine (a CYP1A2) could increase the amount of drug in the blood, but again the implications of this are not known. Somewhat similar to olaparib, there is no strong information on whether this drug is increased, decreased, or not impacted by CBD use. It appears that some studies impacting the metabolism of this drug could also, at least theoretically, be impacted by CBD.

The Near Future—

Other PARP inhibitors being tested now and combination therapies with other CRPC drugs

Additional PARP inhibitors that are approved for use in other cancers and are being studied in prostate cancer include the following:

- **Niraparib** (also known as "Zejula") which is used in certain types of ovarian cancer right now is also being tested in prostate cancer.

- **Talazoparib** (also known as "Talzenna") which is used for certain types of breast cancer right now is also being tested in prostate cancer.

Genetic counselors are a part of some medical teams today, so do not hesitate to call them because they can be very helpful in explaining the results to you and what they may or may not imply for your family/kids in terms of future risk (or no risk).

Please note, if you undergo any genetic testing most reputable companies today offer some form of free consultation with a genetic counselor evaluating your results, including the impact of those results on a variety of family members, especially when doing germline testing. If you are having trouble understanding your germline or somatic test do not hesitate to call the company that completed your test and ask for a genetic counselor to explain the results to you, as well as the potential impact on your kids (if any) or other family members (brothers, sisters, etc.). Additionally, please consult with your direct medical treatment team.

> ### PW Lifestyle Empowerment Moment
>
> There are numerous potential genetic tests out there today, but you should talk to your medical team about which ones are actually "ACTIONABLE," meaning if you are positive for this test, then you (or your family/kids) are at a potential advantage in knowing you have

this biomarker, and can do something about it, compared to other biomarker tests that are "NON-ACTIONABLE." These non-actionable tests can cause a lot of anxiety and expense for arguably no good reason. There are many mutations of interest—just a partial list is provided below. Again, when you are tested, please ask your medical team which mutations or genetic changes are potentially actionable because this can change on a regular basis based on the latest research.

Just for your information, and as an indicator of this growing field of precision medicine, we've listed some of the genes of interest in prostate and/other cancers, and in some cases from germline testing (inherited), or somatic testing:

ATM	MLH1
BRCA1	MSH2
BRCA2	MSH6
BARD1	NBN
BRIP1	PALB2
CDK12	PMS2
CHEK1	RAD51B
CHEK2	RAD51C
EPCAM	RAD51D
FANCL	RAD54L
HOXB13	TP53

Note: *Some genes are associated with a greater risk of being diagnosed with what is known as "Lynch syndrome"—LS (also known as "HNPCC-Hereditary Non-Polyposis Colorectal Cancer"), which is the most common cause of hereditary colorectal cancer. However, somewhat similar to the story of BRCA-1 and BRCA-2 genes, which were thought to be associated with breast and ovarian cancer only and are now associated with multiple cancers including prostate cancer, it appears LS is also associated with a higher risk of multiple cancers (colorectal, ovarian, uterine, adrenal, testicular, stomach, liver, kidney, brain, some forms of skin cancer, etc.), and now even a higher risk of prostate cancer especially with a specific mutation (MSH2). It is autosomal dominant and runs in families often causing a diagnosis of cancer before the age of 50. The five germline mutational or DNA mismatch repair (MMR) genes associated and tested for LS are the following (note: identifying any one or more of the five below are associated with LS):*

- **EPCAM**
- **MLH1**
- **MSH2** (also a higher risk of prostate cancer)
- **MSH6**
- **PMS2**

LS is simply one of the most common hereditary cancer conditions. It is estimated that as high as approximately 1 in 300 people could be carriers of one or some of these gene alterations or mutations. If cancers occurring because of Lynch syndrome can be prevented, or better treated, then there should also be some positive impact on prostate cancer research. For example, exercise is being studied now in Lynch syndrome to see if it can prevent colorectal and perhaps other cancers. Cholesterol controlling medications (statins) are also being studied in a separate clinical trial, as is low-dose and regular strength aspirin based on past preliminary studies showing a potential benefit. There are now similar studies occurring in prostate cancer patients after definitive treatment or with definitive treatment.

Part of the excitement of prostate cancer research today is virtually everything and anything that could be demonstrating some impact against this disease is getting tested. Talk to your medical team about the latest research.

Notes:

_____

_____

_____

_____

_____

_____

_____

_____

_____

_____

_____

_____

_____

_____

_____

_____

_____

_____

_____

_____

_____

_____

CHAPTER 8

Diet, Supplements And Other Lifestyle (Alternative) Options

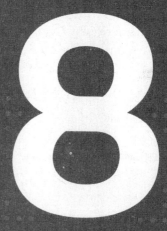

Diet, Supplements, and other Lifestyle (alternative) Options

Every chapter in this book now contains LIFESTYLE EMPOWERMENT MOMENTS but we thought it would be nice to add a few more tips at the end of the book because we believe lifestyle changes can change lives by preventing or alleviating side effects, as well as helping you become more mentally and physically healthy. Though we have also thoroughly discussed numerous treatment options for AdvPCa and suggested methods of dealing with some of the side effects of those treatments, you should rely on your medical team who are experts in preventing and lessening the side effects of your treatments. Be sure to talk to them about your concerns or experiences when dealing with any side effect. Still, it is worth considering some general tips to improve wellness while undergoing treatment, or in many cases, improving overall wellness.

Top Ten Dietary and Lifestyle Recommendations

Tip 1, Part I If you are overweight or concerned about weight gain, a slight reduction in total calories from any food or beverage source is the goal. Keep in mind that reducing just 100 to 200 calories every day can help you to lose weight or maintain your weight. It does not matter where the reduction in the calories occurs—from juices, sugary sodas, half a candy bar, less rice, pasta, or bread...you pick!

Tip 1, Part II If you are underweight or trying to gain weight, a slight increase in total calories from any food or beverage source is the goal. Conversely, increasing your caloric intake daily by just 100 to 200 calories could help with weight gain. You can select the calorie source that you enjoy the most.

Tip 2 Breaking a sweat improves mental and physical health but keep it moderate or it can make things worse. Getting a minimum of 30 minutes a day of movement time is a great tool to improve mental as well as physical health. However, during cancer treatment try to limit extensive or intense aerobic workouts to not more than every other day as opposed to daily because that activity level can increase fatigue. Your body takes longer to recover from a workout when there is less testosterone in your system and during cancer treatment in general, so exercising every day can make you more tired. You should work with your medical team to determine how vigorous your exercise program should be. Be sure to check with your medical team to see how best to incorporate exercise into your routine.

Tip 3 Weightlifting or resistance exercise just twice a week has diverse mental and physical health benefits. Ask your medical team if you can do upper and/or lower body weightlifting two or three times a week for 15 to 30 minutes each time. If it is possible, this can stimulate muscle growth, increase your metabolism, burn belly fat, reduce fatigue, reduce the risk of bone loss, and improve mental health during cancer treatment. If you are not allowed to lift weights because of your bone metastasis, try to do some light resistance exercise by doing swimming pool aerobics, walking, doing tai chi, or any other exercise that requires some movement and a little pressure on the muscles and bones. Additionally, socialized exercise or exercising with a group, friend, spouse etc., appears to offer quality of life benefits beyond working out by yourself.

Tip 4 Keep your cardiovascular disease risk as close to zero as possible. Most heart-healthy changes have an anti–prostate cancer effect. It is a fact that too many men with AdvPCa die every year from heart disease, the number one overall cause of death in men. Therefore, considering heart health makes sense for everyone, including AdvPCa patients. LDL ("bad cholesterol") should be below 100 minimally, HDL ("good cholesterol") as high above 40 as possible, and triglycerides less than 100. Try to monitor your hs-CRP level to keep it low, and your blood pressure should stay within a normal range. It is interesting that virtually everything found to be heart healthy (exercise, weight loss, low cholesterol, low blood pressure) has turned out to have some anti–prostate cancer impact. If that weren't enough, another reason to follow your heart-healthy numbers is that they provide some real proof that any lifestyle change you are making is providing a benefit. For example, changing your diet or exercise can lower cholesterol, blood pressure, and blood sugar, reduce waist size, and provides evidence to you that the changes you are making are helping you.

Tip 5 Healthy fats and less liquid sugar, please! Consume healthy fats, such as monounsaturated and polyunsaturated (Omega-3) fats, which come from healthy sources, such as fatty fish, lean meat, nuts, plant oils, and seeds. Minimize saturated fat intake, in some cases, not because it is unhealthy, but because most foods and beverages with higher amounts of saturated fat simply contain an excess of calories. You can select nearly identical beverages and foods and simply choose the one lower in saturated fat and/or calories. Think about milk for a second: almond, soy, flax, and skim milk often contain no saturated fat and deliver 25 to 80 calories or fewer for an 8-ounce serving, but 2% and whole milk contain almost twice as many calories in the same serving! Liquid sugar or carbohydrates, from fruit juice to soda to alcohol, in excess contribute too many calories and can make it very easy to gain weight.

Tip 6 Consume 20 to 30 grams of fiber a day, but not from pills or commercialized powders. Insoluble fiber and small amounts of soluble fiber (the two types of fiber) come from bran cereal, chia seed, flaxseed, lentils and beans, and low-calorie fruits and vegetables. Fiber helps prevent acid reflux, constipation, weight gain, and it lowers blood pressure, cholesterol, and even PSA in some studies. However, do not rely on fiber pills and powders for the majority of your fiber intake because they are much more expensive than fiber from food, contain mostly soluble fiber that can upset your stomach, and require enormous intakes to reach your 20 to 30 grams a day requirement. Did you know that most commercial fiber pills require anywhere from 10 to 60 capsules a day to reach your recommended daily allowance? No kidding! As an alternative, try just 1/3 cup of Bran Buds cereal with a little flaxseed and fruit to provide 20 grams of fiber. As an added bonus, it will cost you very little!

Tip 7 The more you process food, the less the nutritional value and the more the calories! Think of any food in its natural state, for example, an apple. An apple is low in calories and high in fiber, but eating applesauce or drinking apple juice means you consume more calories (and sugar) and little or no fiber. Generally, fruit and some vegetable juices are high-calorie inadequate substitutes for the real thing. Whole-grain bread, or even simple wheat bread, has better nutritional and fiber value as compared to plain white bread. Grass-fed beef has less saturated fat, more healthy fats, and just as much protein as less nutritious grain-fed or frozen patties of beef. Plain yogurt (or even plain Greek yogurt) is more nutritious and contains fewer calories as compared to flavored yogurt or yogurt-flavored drinks. In other words, whenever possible try to pick foods that have not been processed to reduce your calories and increase your nutritional health benefits.

Tip 8 Sodium from the saltshaker is not the problem, but potassium is the answer. Salt or sodium in excess can raise blood pressure. The recommended intake of 2400 mg per day to lower blood pressure can readily be achieved by reducing sodium from processed foods (check labels and pick the food that is lower in sodium). In reality, salt from the saltshaker is only a minor contributor to the total. In fact, in one of the most famous studies in the world (DASH), reducing sodium intake to 1500 mg or less along with diet changes and exercise provided results equivalent to most blood pressure medications. Using small amounts of seasonings and spices is a great way to get more flavor from your food without using excess salt.

Regardless, diets low in sodium are generally high in potassium, magnesium, and other healthy nutrients such as protein and fiber (think beans, fish, fruits, vegetables, nuts, plain yogurt, and seeds). High potassium-based foods naturally allow you to eat healthier and potassium is arguably one of the only major nutrients not being consumed at anywhere near the recommended or adequate intake (approximately 2600 mg for adult women and 3400 mg per day for men).

Potassium-Rich Foods	Amount of Potassium mg/serving
Salmon	628
Beans	561
Leafy dark greens	558
Baked potato (w/skin)	535
Figs	500
Avocado	485
Acorn squash	437
Mushrooms	396
Bananas	358
Yogurt	255

Tip 9 The "sin foods" or beverages are not the issue, and they may actually be beneficial. Alcohol, chocolate, ice cream, coffee, meat...oh my! These things must be bad for you! Not really! In excess they are not heart healthy, but in moderation they can make you feel better and serve as a wonderful reward for following healthy lifestyle changes most of the time. In other words, maintaining a sense of normalcy is critical to maintaining overall mental and physical health. One diet that has documented success is the Mediterranean diet. Research suggests that it has numerous health benefits as compared to other diet programs. If you look over the list of foods included in the Mediterranean diet, you'll find a diversity of healthy foods and beverages. It also promotes "everything in moderation" and includes foods and beverages that are not necessarily healthy for you. It appears

that consuming more foods in moderation leads to more success than consuming several things in excess. It is also interesting that the Mediterranean diet does not involve taking a lot of dietary supplements or any other pills to prevent health problems.

Also worth noting is that many cancer books in the past suggested that coffee and caffeine were bad for you, but now clinical research suggests that consuming some caffeine from beverages can not only improve liver function, but also reduce fatigue and have anticancer effects. It may also prevent other diseases, improve mental health, and enhance muscle recovery after workouts. However, in megadoses or when caffeine is taken from a pill, the concentrated form can increase heart rate and blood pressure and is not heart healthy.

Tip 10 Stress, anxiety, depression, lack of sleep, and other issues that impact your mental health are also bad for your physical health. "Whatever it takes"—this should be your motto when it comes to mental health. You must make sure that your mental health is as much of a priority as your physical health, and you should do whatever is needed to get there. Stress can dramatically increase your level of certain hormones that could have a negative impact on some cancer treatments. Stress can cause the release of abnormally high amounts of inflammatory substances and other compounds that can suppress your immune system, cause heart-unhealthy changes, and make it difficult to sleep and relax. If depression, stress, or anxiety is an issue, please seek professional assistance, counseling, more social support—whatever else is needed.

Supplements/Other CAM/OTC/RX

The vast array of dietary supplements can make you dizzy. It seems that every day we hear about some "new benefit" of taking certain supplements, and in some cases, new warnings. How do you know which supplements are truly beneficial and which ones to avoid? The same is true of over the counter (OTC) medications, prescriptions, and complementary and alternative medicine (CAM). For instance, acupuncture is receiving a lot of positive attention for helping cancer patients. Does it really work?

This section attempts to answer these questions, and more, while providing the latest information on a wide range of supplements and other common drugs, as well as CAM. As you can see from the length of this section, there is a lot of information to cover! In addition to this book, we recommend the following comprehensive websites to learn more. Please do your research!

Best FREE Websites on Supplements (Top 3, in no particular order, from my world, but there are many others.)

You get what you pay for? Not always! Check out these three outstanding FREE websites to stay current on the latest, greatest, and not so great dietary supplements and other complementary and alternative medicines (CAM) along with plenty of medical references. These evidence-based websites are updated on a regular basis. (Note: NIH stands for National Institutes of Health, which is a U.S. government agency.)

NIH Office of Dietary Supplements (ODS)

ods.od.nih.gov

This site includes "Dietary Supplement Fact Sheets" from A-to-Z (in English & Spanish). They are concise, easy to read, and just as easy to access. Additionally, they try to include a table of the top food sources of the nutrient being discussed. I love it!

NIH National Center for Complementary & Integrative Health (NCCIH)

nccih.nih.gov

This site includes "Health Topics A-Z," or "Herbs at a glance." Simply type in the supplement or complementary medicine of interest and bam! It's a great resource for updated general, CAM, and specific supplement information. I love it!

"About Herbs" Website and Phone App from the Memorial Sloan Kettering Cancer Center (MSKCC)

mskcc.org (Type in "about herbs" on their website and it will take you where you need to go)

You'll find over 200 monographs on supplements (pros, cons, studies, drug interactions, etc.), and you can also download the free "About Herbs App" for your phone. This is one of the best websites in the world for cancer patients looking to get the best and latest information on a variety of supplement options and non-options, and other CAM including mind-body therapies. Even if you're not dealing with cancer the updated and comprehensive information provided on this site is outstanding. I love it (but you knew I would say that)!

The Clean (never dirty) Dozen—Quick tips before taking any supplement, CAM, or pill

1. Before any medical treatment be one with your healthcare team.

Healthcare teams and medical organizations are becoming more educated daily on supplements and CAM. So, please talk to your healthcare team before taking any supplement or trying any CAM. Keep in mind, your team may include your pharmacist, nutritionist, and others who can provide the latest and greatest and not so great information on any supplement. Also, approximately 2-3 weeks before any surgical, radiation or other prostate cancer procedure or treatment, please review the dietary supplements you are using with your healthcare team to determine which ones are safe to take during this time. You don't want some supplement to interact with your anesthesia or blood thinners, mitigate the impact of radiation, or increase the side effects of chemotherapy or another treatment option.

On the other hand, some supplements look interesting as an option to reduce the side effects of some cancer treatments, such as calcium and vitamin D (if not able to get adequate amounts from dietary sources) when on a bone mineral density drug (BMD) for androgen deprivation treatment (ADT), or L-citrulline along with standard prescription treatments for erectile dysfunction (ED). So having this conversation is a win-win situation.

2. Biotin (vitamin B7)—Blurry lab results are possible (aka "biotin interference").

Individual biotin supplements could be a problem if taken several days before your PSA and other blood tests. Biotin supplements (especially in large amounts) have an ability to interfere with the accuracy of some blood tests (assays) by potentially causing false elevations, or reductions, in some blood tests. If you're taking biotin, it's best to stop several days before your next blood test and be sure to tell your healthcare team you're taking it. Today most laboratory companies have formally recognized this phenomenon and have placed warnings on the specific tests most likely to encounter "biotin interference."

3. DILI & HILI needs LFT attention ASAP ("herbals are a different animal").

Drug induced liver injury (DILI) is a growing major problem. Not long ago a tiny percentage of DILI was caused by supplements, while the vast majority was due to prescription drugs. Recently, the percentage of DILI caused by dietary supplements has been estimated to be as high as 20% (1 out of 5) of the cases! For this, and other reasons, herbal induced liver injury (HILI) is now becoming an accepted part of DILI, since some herbals, especially fly-by-night products have been more concerning than others in terms of drug interactions and their impact on the liver. "Herbals are a different animal" is another one of my teaching mantras because so many compounds from similar or different parts of the plant (leaf, root, stem, etc.) and potential contaminants could be inside some herbal products, due to the way the product is sourced. Therefore, it generally requires more homework on your part when looking for a clean product (also see the third-party piece of advice/table later in this chapter). Another good solution is to always work with your healthcare team to monitor your liver enzymes and other tests when you start any product to see if you develop a problem. Performing liver function tests (LFTs) is done all the time for drugs such as abiraterone, which has a higher risk of liver toxicity.

4. Generalizing extreme amounts of negativity or positivity never helps supplements or drugs.

Some "experts" love to say everything good or bad about dietary supplements and this makes little sense to me. Supplements, like drugs, should not be generalized as an entire category in terms of clinical evidence, but should stand on their own merit for the specific condition being discussed. For example, the widespread acceptance of melatonin as a supplement or prescription in lower dosages is impressive. However, when some paint with a broad brush claiming they have no value, while others argue they work for everyone, then both these misunderstood generalizations are not only inaccurate, but also harmful to improving dietary supplement education for patients and health care professionals (HCP).

Melatonin is one of the primary treatment options for REM sleep behavior disorder—a serious condition, which not only could be dangerous to the person experiencing it, but also their partner sleeping next to them. In addition, the American Academy of Pediatrics (AAP) thinks melatonin is a potential insomnia treatment option in lower dosages for some children with autism spectrum disorder (ASD), and there are suggestions it can help some cancer patients with sleeping difficulties. Although, the idea currently that it treats cancer, including prostate cancer sounds impressive, studies have not been impressive thus far, but more are scheduled to be completed soon. Also, it's not safe for many people to take large dosages of melatonin because of the potential for certain drug interactions, changes in hormones, and other more serious side effects.

5. Inactive ingredients could still be quite active in some individuals.

Research suggests many pills (both medications and supplements) are made up of a greater proportion of inactive ingredients (75%) compared to active ingredients (25%). This is often necessary to improve stability, solubility, taste, and other consumer friendly reasons. Yet, some of these inactive ingredients could be "active" or problematic for certain individuals, so always check the list. For example, one of the more common inactive ingredients is lactose, which could be a problem if you're lactose intolerant. A person could also be sensitive to other compounds such as certain dyes on the inactive ingredient list. If you think you could be sensitive to any of these ingredients, or if you think you've already had a reaction to one or more of the inactive ingredients then please talk to your healthcare team and the manufacturer about the specific dosage of the inactive ingredient in the product. You will almost always have the option of switching brands and still getting the same active ingredient, but without the inactive ingredient of concern to you.

6. "Less is always more" until you really know if you absolutely need more (aka "take nothing until you know you need something").

"Take nothing until you know you need something" is another mantra I teach because it's better to be safe than sorry before spending money on something ineffective or dangerous. There is probably no better example of "less is more" in medicine than in prostate cancer where several supplements could encourage the growth of some tumors. For example, one study (the SELECT trial) found that vitamin E in higher supplemental doses can have this effect. Decades ago, these same supplements were touted to help fight prostate cancer in mega dosages, but without strong evidence. Other examples include products that increase testosterone and adrenal hormones (e.g., DHEA). While these products may be okay for some men and women, they could have the ability to stimulate tumor growth in prostate cancer patients. Again, less is more until you know for sure you need more!

7. Look for a third party to join your party.

One of the common criticisms of supplements is the lack of proven quality control in some (not all) instances. However, this has changed dramatically today with the addition of numerous organizations testing and/or simply reporting on the quality control (OC) of many brands. A partial list of sites to check can be found in the following table.

(**Note:** *This is only a partial listing of all the high-quality reporting on supplements available. Some cost money and others do not, but these are examples of why the situation is getting better in terms of QC and reporting accuracy. For example, BSCG, NSF, USP, UL, and others are some of the QC seals you want to see listed on a website or products from a supplement sales site. Just one of these QC symbols or certificates is often adequate on a website or supplement bottle. Some of the sites listed below are more well-known for objective information on health and supplements, such as Consumer Reports or CSPI.)*

Examples of PW Quality Control (QC) Groups known to test and/or regularly report on the efficacy and safety of dietary supplements from A-to-Z	Websites for More Information and Commentary
Aegis Shield	aegisshield.com
Banned Substances Control Group (BSCG)	bscg.org
Center for Science in the Public Interest (CSPI)	cspi.org
Consumer Labs	consumerlab.com

Consumer Reports (magazine, digital, and health newsletter)	consumerreports.org
Eurofins	eurofins.com
Informed-Choice/Informed Sport	informed-sport.com
ISURA (Isura)	isura.ca
NSF International	nsf.org
Tested to be Trusted (CVS pharmacy now has supplements tested with some of these QC groups)	CVS pharmacy or others (Ask your pharmacy/supplement seller anywhere you live in the world if they have supplement QC standards)
UL (Underwriters Laboratories)	ul.com
USP (United States Pharmacopeia Convention)	usp.org

Note: *The FDA and Health Canada also provide supplement safety alerts, concerns, and information. Isura is currently Canada's only independent, not-for-profit supplement and food verification and certification group. The above list works for some countries, such as the U.S. and Canada, but you and your healthcare team can create your own list wherever you live in the world. Patients and their healthcare teams should always inquire about a Certificate of Analysis (COA) or more proof of QC.*

8. Only as good and safe as your last update ("it's just good medicine to regularly check on the efficacy and safety of your medicines").

This is a simple rule. Supplements are getting more research now than at any other point in human history, which means you could wake up one day and find that your specific supplements are not as safe, or perhaps safer than they were a year or even a month before. Always check on the latest pros, cons, drug interactions, and any other new research on the product you're thinking about using. This is also true for any drug you're taking or medical intervention you're considering because of the incredible amounts of global research going on in every aspect of medicine. "It's just good medicine to regularly check on the safety and efficacy of your medicines!" (Sorry, another one of my teaching mantras that I could never get out of my cranium during lectures to my colleagues and patient advocacy groups.)

9. RDA is making you feel guilty? Then focus on your EAR and watch your pill count decrease!

The so-called "recommended daily allowance" (RDA) is a bit of a misnomer or misunderstood phrase that can lead to extra pill taking for many nutrients, such as calcium, vitamin D, B12, etc. The RDA appears to make many folks think this is the level of intake they need to achieve on average, or what they should aim for every day. Cue the incorrect buzzer sound! Some people think if they cannot achieve the RDA then they need to make up the rest in supplements of that specific nutrient. Cue the incorrect buzzer sound again! The reality is the more important concept of the "estimated average requirement" (EAR) has not received enough attention. The lesser-known EAR is, in general, the most likely or more appropriate nutrient requirement for approximately 97.5% of the population. Meanwhile, the RDA is the potential nutrient consumption needs for people at the far end of the population curve – meaning virtually everyone in a population will have nutrient needs BELOW THE RDA! The RDA helps to cover those at the more extreme ends of the population in terms of a nutrient needs. Yes, there are some situations and conditions that place some folks at that end, but most people need far less than the RDA, and need to shoot for the EAR (sounds pugilistic, but it's not)!

When you see an RDA or any other nutrient requirement, always check how the EAR compares. Often, you'll find it to be lower and more manageable in terms of dietary intake and only rarely will you need to make up the rest in terms of supplements. However, if your healthcare team thinks you need to shoot for the RDA, then please follow their advice. In general, most of us should be happy with the EAR! Calcium, vitamin D, and countless other nutrients have an EAR lower than the RDA. For example, if you take what is known as a "thiazide diuretic" for your blood pressure it could lead to greater absorption of calcium into the body (decreases urinary calcium loss), so taking the RDA of vitamin D and calcium in this case could cause too much exposure! On the other hand, being on androgen deprivation therapy (ADT), or taking prednisone could increase your calcium and vitamin D needs because both medications accelerate bone loss (reduce absorption and processing of these nutrients), so you may need to aim for the RDA. In this book, we like to recommend the numerical range from the EAR to the RDA (not just the RDA alone), but not more than that unless you fall into a special category of need based on the experience of your healthcare team and not some book (like this one).

10. Perception vs. Reality? Pick the reality of the specific medical condition and then the reality in other areas of medicine.

Like many drugs, supplements could be beneficial in one area of medicine, and not so beneficial in another area. Some of the discouraged supplements or medications within prostate cancer are one reality, but outside of this medical condition these products may be helpful, harmful, or do nothing (a different reality). For example, individual vitamin E supplements are generally discouraged in prostate cancer, but they have a role as part of a combination supplement for age-related macular degeneration from the well-known AREDS trials. In other words, just because a product looks good or bad for prostate cancer does not suggest it could be harmful or beneficial outside of cancer, so always check with your healthcare team before adding or subtracting anything from your supplement list. This is also true for prescription medications such as beta-blockers, which could be helpful in multiple different areas of medicine (e.g., cardiovascular, migraine, etc.), but for individuals with certain types of lung issues, such as asthma, they could be harmful. Countless drugs look great in one area and worthless or even harmful in another area of medicine. The secret is determining when the pros exceed the cons, or when the cons exceed the pros for your situation or condition(s).

11. Supplements are prescription drugs in many countries (perception vs. reality part two).

Melatonin and melatonin receptor agonists (which bind to the receptor) are prescription drugs in the U.S. and around the world. But wait, aren't they also supplements? Yes! Some of the biggest selling supplements have a prescription option in the same place or another location around the globe. For example, fish oil or even some amino acid supplements such as L-glutamine both have a supplement and prescription option in the U.S. This is another reason not to get misguided by the idea that supplements (when effective) are much different from a drug and vice versa. The reality is an effective supplement is a drug, which it is not necessarily a bad thing, but it's concerning when some folks consider an effective supplement safer or better than a drug in the same category, which is more of a perception.

12. Supplement users like heart healthy lifestyles and personal empowerment vs. just pill taking. (Perception vs. reality part three.)

When lecturing to healthcare professionals (HCPs), I often remind them that research continues to demonstrate that patients, and even HCPs, who are interested in or taking supplements are more likely to embrace and follow heart healthy lifestyle changes. The perception of people who take supplements needs to change in some circles because this is a group that demonstrates a strong affinity toward improving lifestyle, and not just letting the pill do all the work. I wish more people would realize this research-based truth. In fact, in the Physicians' Healthy Study 2 (PHS2), which was one of the largest and best randomized trials in the supplement world, found that the physicians using supplements before and during the study were more likely to be healthier and sensitive to making lifestyle changes!

One more point to remember is when your own 5Bs get better, then it appears blood levels of many nutrients can increase, such as vitamin D or 25-OH vitamin D. In other words, as you become healthier via your lifestyle then fewer pills or smaller dosages of supplements may be needed because these pills work better or more efficiently at a healthier weight (hey, just like many prescription drugs, and even some vaccines have been more effective in healthier weight individuals from past studies). In fact, the VITAL trial of vitamin D from Harvard appeared to demonstrate greater efficacy of vitamin D supplementation for prevention of several different health outcomes when carrying a healthier weight (body mass index)!

Supplements/Other CAM/OTC/RX and Diet from A-Z

Note: Before we begin this section, please remember there is a concern with multiple supplements having the ability to promote prostate cancer growth, so when in doubt "less is more." In addition, other specific supplements used to reduce the side effects of some cancer treatments have both negative and positive data and should be discussed individually with your healthcare team. Finally, keep in mind this section is loaded with PW Lifestyle Empowerment Moments throughout, so we decided to not call them out except at the end of this chapter. As you will see, PW pill-less options or lifestyle empowerment is a large part of this section!

Acetaminophen (e.g., paracetamol or Tylenol)— Liver and new BP issues.

Higher dosages of acetaminophen, especially combined with alcohol can cause liver toxicity (it is still one of the most common causes of acute liver failure), and it has demonstrated no consistent impact (either good or bad) on prostate cancer (neutral effect). In addition, although it was once believed that these drugs did not impact blood pressure, recent evidence suggests larger daily dosages of acetaminophen could raise systolic blood pressure (BP) in some patients with hypertension (treated or untreated). So be careful, especially since acetaminophen is an ingredient in so many medications, including cold and flu formulas, muscle, headache, and other pain relievers. This is one of the reasons people inadvertently take too much acetaminophen. Other potential recent side effects attributed to higher dosages of acetaminophen, such as kidney function and gastrointestinal bleeding, need more research for clarity.

Acetyl-L-Carnitine and chemotherapy do not mix right now.

The American Society of Clinical Oncology (ASCO), which is one of the most reputable oncology groups in the world, published a recent clinical guideline update on how to treat chemotherapy induced peripheral neuropathy (CIPN), which is nerve injury weakness or numbness in the hands and/or feet. In this publication they discouraged the use of the supplement acetyl-L-carnitine (ALC) for the prevention of CIPN. This advice needs to be taken seriously because it's based on clinical research suggesting it could do more harm than good. CIPN can be caused by prostate cancer chemotherapy, and you want to ensure nothing is done to discourage the recovery from the condition or make it worse. This is a case where a supplement should not be used to prevent or treat this side effect from some cancer treatments. Interestingly, acupuncture, exercise and keeping some of the 5 Bs healthy have been associated with a lower risk or severity of CIPN!

Acid Reflux Medications, B12, and many lifestyle options are also groovy.

Over the counter (OTC) and prescription acid reflux medications have an ability to reduce blood levels of vitamin B12 and magnesium in some patients. If you've been taking, or are taking these medications on a regular basis, then please ask your healthcare team about getting a vitamin B12 blood test just to make sure everything is okay. Then ask if you also need an occasional magnesium test. Long-term use of acid reflux medications (H2 blockers, PPIs-Proton Pump Inhibitors, etc.) have been tied to many nutrient reductions and absorption problems but decreases in B12 is the more widely agreed upon issue. (Please see the B12 section in this chapter because many things can cause a low B12 level.) Also, please keep in mind weight loss, sleeping on your left side, increased intake of dietary fiber, smaller meals, and reducing or eliminating some of the trigger foods/beverages are just some of the many lifestyle changes that could improve your acid reflux (GERD) symptoms, whether taking medicine or not for this condition.

Acupuncture/Acupressure is getting more positive attention, and it may reduce some pill dosages and counts.

There is preliminary evidence that acupuncture can be beneficial within prostate cancer, as well as urology and general oncology. These finding are summarized in the table below.

Acupuncture—Potential Benefit in Prostate Cancer/Urology	Commentary
Reduced frequency and/or severity of androgen deprivation therapy (ADT) side effects, including hot flashes/flushes/night sweats (commonly called "vasomotor symptoms")	One of the only medical treatments in which safety concerns are minimal and preliminary overall impact is consistently positive (reduces hot flashes), but more sham (placebo) acupuncture comparison groups and larger studies of longer duration are needed.
Alleviates some cancer medication/treatment induced discomfort	Acupuncture and acupressure have preliminary positive data in this area including reducing discomfort (arthralgia and myalgia) caused by some cancer medications/treatments.
Reduced chemotherapy side effects, including chemotherapy-induced peripheral neuropathy (CIPN)	Few safe or even proven effective options exist for CIPN, but preliminary data suggests a reduction in neuropathic pain even beyond what is observed with sham acupuncture.
Alleviates Chronic Prostatitis (CP)/Chronic Pelvic Pain Syndrome (CPPS) and other potential urologic-associated pain syndromes such as IC/BPS (interstitial cystitis/bladder pain syndrome)	Urologic pain syndrome improvements are a promising area of research to reduce or avoid the impact on unnecessary or addiction provoking medications.

Calms overactive bladder (OAB) (Urge incontinence)	A form of electro-acupuncture is already a standard of care (PTNS; for example, Medtronic, Urgent PC®, etc.), especially for some patients not responding to or unable to tolerate the standard prescription medicines for this condition. Other forms of acupuncture also hold promise.

Note: *BPH and sexual dysfunction (ED) lack reliable consistent data and need more research. Other acute or chronic pain urologic and non-urologic clinical situations would be interesting to research, which, if beneficial, could reduce addiction potential or dependency, or reduce dosages of some pain medications.*

Aspirin and the Add-Aspirin Phase 3 Trial (addaspirintrial.org)— Wait and see please.

Aspirin is used in many individuals for the secondary prevention of a cardiovascular event such as preventing another heart attack or ischemic stroke. It has shown some promise in reducing the risk of certain cancers, but it has also been associated with an increased risk of internal bleeding and ulcers, especially in patients that do not qualify for it. Aspirin is being tested in a phase 3 trial known as "Add-Aspirin" to determine if it could reduce the risk of prostate and other cancer (e.g., breast, colorectal, esophageal, stomach) recurrence after conventional treatment. The results of this trial should be available soon. See addaspirintrial.org for more information. In the meantime, the only reason to go on low-dose or regular aspirin is because you qualify for it based on your cardiovascular risk history. A large recent randomized study of regular aspirin (300 mg/day) in breast cancer (Aspirin after Breast Cancer, or ABC trial) to prevent recurrence did not work better than placebo. But will it work in prostate or other cancers after treatment? Ask your healthcare team about the latest results please.

Ashwagandha, DHEA, Fenugreek Seed Extract, Tongkat Ali, Tribulus Terrestris, and other potential DHEAS and/or testosterone increasing products do not mix with BPH or prostate cancer right now.

Please avoid these supplements if you have been diagnosed with prostate cancer because the adrenal hormone DHEAS, for example, could be increased by some of these products, which could potentially stimulate prostate tumor growth. In addition, there is some preliminary research suggesting they could also increase prostate size. The DHEA, DHEAS, or testosterone increasing category of supplements may look good for some other situations, but it's best to avoid them if you've been diagnosed with prostate cancer, and/or BPH. In fact, some of the companies selling these products have already done a good job of mentioning these concerns on their website, or in another location. There has been a lot of discussion over whether some men should be on any testosterone replacement treatment (TRT), especially a prescription form of this drug, after being successfully treated or considered cured of their prostate cancer for some time. However, a discussion of the pros and cons should never be handled by a book, but rather a conversation with your healthcare team.

B12—Be aware that deficiency/insufficiency can occur. Low cost may be as good as the expensive options.

Ask your healthcare team to test your blood at some point to see if you have adequate B12 levels, or if you need to boost your intake of foods with B12 or take a B12 supplement. B12 comes from animal food sources (for example, salmon) and fortified products, but acid reflux medications, metformin, plant-based diets, autoimmune gastritis, surgical removal of part of the small intestine (ileum) for example in some patients (cystectomy with urinary diversion utilizing ileum), weight gain or loss, and other situations could have a significant impact on reducing your blood levels of B12. B12 has not been shown to fight prostate cancer, and excessive amounts are not helpful either, but low B12 levels can create all sorts of symptoms that could mimic other diseases and reduce quality of life.

There is also a widespread belief that more potentially expensive B12 injections are needed when absorption of B12 is compromised. This is not correct in some cases because the entire intestinal tract (not just the ileum) absorbs a tiny amount of B12 by passive diffusion from low-cost supplements. In fact, in head-to-head studies, the low cost B12 option worked as well as the more costly injections over time for many individuals.

Biotin (also known as vitamin B7) supplements in high dosages can cause false increases or decreases in some important blood tests.

This topic, already mentioned at the beginning of this chapter, needs to be repeated. Taking mega-dosages of some supplements can artificially change the results of some laboratory tests. For example, mega-dosages of vitamin C and E could alter the results of a hemoglobin A1c (blood sugar) test, also mentioned earlier in the book. This is another of the many reasons why it's important to talk to your healthcare team before taking any supplements. They should know exactly what you're taking and in what dosage so they can help you prevent these things from happening. Individual B7 supplements increasing the risk of altering lab test results is a newer phenomenon, but the lab companies are adding warnings to many blood tests, as well as making sure some of their tests do not interfere with this supplement.

BPH drugs (finasteride & dutasteride) and/or BPH supplements—and don't forget those similar, but often lower dose prescription hair drugs!

Saw palmetto was in two major clinical trials in the U.S./North America known as "STEP" and "CAMUS." Both trials failed to demonstrate a benefit of saw palmetto compared to placebo for BPH. However, a European prescription form or regulated brand of saw palmetto known as "Permixon" continues to accumulate positive data. How could this be the case? If you favor saw palmetto one could argue the fatty acid and sterol content of Permixon is unique because of their isolation or extraction method (hexane-based) compared to the products used in STEP (CO_2 extraction) and CAMUS (ethanolic extraction method). On the other hand, one could argue that the European product needs more head-to-head research and against a better placebo. Regardless, two things are known: Saw palmetto appears to be as safe as a placebo, so some men and their physicians like it; but there is no strong evidence it has any activity to prevent or treat prostate cancer.

There are two BPH drugs known as finasteride or dutasteride which can shrink larger prostates and help prevent the progression of BPH. However, these drugs have some controversy attached to them because they can reduce ejaculate volume, impact sexual function, and there have been some reports of other not so pleasant side effects. These drugs are expected to reduce PSA by approximately 50%, but do they reduce the risk of low-grade prostate cancer? They appear to have some impact, but do not reduce the risk of high-grade cancer, or lower the risk of dying from prostate cancer. Still, if PSA increases while on these drugs it's often a sign that the person taking them needs to be evaluated to see if prostate cancer is causing that increase since often the BPH is being controlled. Thus, although these drugs carry some controversy with them, they also carry some benefit when needed. This is a classic example of why individualized care is so critical.

Less well known is the fact that lower dose versions of these drugs are used throughout the world to prevent male pattern baldness and they have helped some men (especially 1 mg finasteride—also known as "Propecia"). However, what needs more immediate attention is the fact that these drugs, even at lower dosages, also reduce PSA by approximately 50%, which means patients taking these drugs need to tell their physicians they are taking one of these drugs and need to be monitored. If PSA increases while on these specific lower dose hair loss drugs there needs to be some investigation as to the cause or reason (e.g., cancer, BPH progression). It should also be known that these drugs could impact male fertility and have been associated with a variety of other side effects, so please talk to your medical team about the latest updates.

There are also a host of BPH supplements claiming to prevent or treat BPH, such as beta-sitosterol or pumpkin seed oil/extract, and although there is some positive data for them more recent rigorous research is needed. Your healthcare team can monitor you when on these or other supplements for your own safety, and they can help you determine if they are effective enough for your situation. Pygeum africanum is another supplement in the BPH area, but there are some environmental controversies with certain sources of these ingredients. Check and see if the companies are using endangered or non-endangered derived options. Regardless, all these BPH supplements have something in common, which is they don't have any strong evidence they impact the risk or progression of prostate cancer.

Calcium and/or Vitamin D3 supplements IF (that is a BIG IF) you cannot get enough from your diet and there is more in the diet than ever before! Please be careful! Most people do not need calcium pills and could be increasing their risk of numerous medical problems by overexposing themselves to excessive amounts of calcium (constipation, stones, cardiovascular, etc.)! First, please remember getting too much calcium from supplements can increase the risk of constipation and/or kidney stones—especially calcium carbonate in terms of stones, but any calcium in excess can increase the risk of constipation. On the other hand, too little calcium, or vitamin D, can increase the risk of bone loss. Recommended daily intakes is usually 1,000-1,200 mg/day of calcium and 600 IU/day of vitamin D up to the age of 70 years and then 800 IU/day from age 71 and older. Most men can get these amounts from foods and beverages or fortified products in the diet, or by simply taking just a single daily multivitamin. Preliminary studies have suggested there are higher amounts of vitamin D in wild-caught salmon compared to farmed salmon, but omega-3 content is often similar between the two options. Today, a wide variety of foods/beverages are fortified with calcium and vitamin D in many countries, including the U.S. For example, most plant-based milks are fortified with calcium and vitamin D (more than dairy in many cases). Many types of fish are good sources of vitamin D, although they are not a great source of calcium—unless you like to eat the bones! Some mushrooms are also good sources of vitamin D when exposed to ultraviolet light by some companies. Be sure to check the labels.

When it comes to supplements, keep in mind that excessive amounts of vitamin D can also increase your risk of high or unhealthy calcium levels in the blood and urine, which could lead to many problems (not just kidney stones). However, the VITAL prevention trial demonstrated that vitamin D3 (2000 IU/day) may have the ability to reduce the risk of autoimmune disease in some people. In the area of cancer, there is not enough data right now to suggest that vitamin D has any impact, except perhaps in people with a healthy BMI (also from the VITAL trial). We need more data before any firm conclusion can be drawn regarding cancer patients. Some would argue that getting more sun is the way to increase vitamin D, but dietary and supplementary sources are easier and safer – and losing just a little weight can also increase your vitamin D blood level. A little sun is okay, but a lot of sun can cause premature wrinkling and increases your risk of skin cancer. If you're vegan, vitamin D2 is an alternative option to vitamin D3, but a new option is vitamin D3 derived from algae!

Calcium supplements come in a variety of types, so make sure you talk with your healthcare team before deciding on the best form needed (i.e., carbonate, citrate, phosphate, etc.). Calcium citrate tends to be a better choice for those with a history of kidney stones, and it can be taken with or without food. Calcium carbonate is a more concentrated option, but it needs to be taken with food for better absorption, and it's also the primary ingredient found in many OTC heartburn relief remedies. Therefore, people with frequent heartburn or reflux issues may already be getting more than enough calcium carbonate. Calcium phosphate should be taken with food and can be found in many multivitamins.

There is also growing evidence that a heart healthy lifestyle reduces bone loss suggesting a variety of other healthy nutrients in the diet (less dietary sodium, more dietary potassium, etc.) can help keep bones healthy! Please look at the table to see how easy it is to eat healthier and get the calcium (or vitamin D) needed without taking extra pills! Many people do NOT need calcium supplements/pills today and could be increasing the risk of numerous medical problems by overexposing themselves to calcium. For example, not just kidney stones and constipation, but they could be heart unhealthy in excess. We are waiting for more research on this so talk to your team about the latest concerns.

Healthy calcium dietary (not pill) sources	Calcium Amount (per single serving) (Age 18 to 70 = 1000 & age 71+ = 1200)
Plant-Based Milks (fortified)	300-500 mg
Coffee with plant milk (soy, etc.)	300-400 mg
Yogurt-plain-Greek, etc.	200-300 mg
Bok Choy, Collard greens, Spinach	100-200 mg
Tofu	100-150 mg
Beans, Lentils, Nuts, or Seeds	50-150 mg
Broccoli, Edamame, Kale,	50-100 mg
Fiber-enriched cereal products	50-100 mg
Oatmeal	50-100 mg
Berries, Figs, Kiwi, Oranges	50-100 mg
Salmon, canned, "boneless"	50 mg (vs. 250 mg "with bones")

Note: *Real milk and other traditional dairy products often contain approximately 300 mg of calcium per serving. Also, some companies are combining several different leafy green veggies, such as baby bok choy, baby kale or spinach in one package/container to increase the nutritional content per serving, which is a fabulous idea!*

CBD—Cannabidiol)/marijuana sounds good, but price, QC (COA is needed), and safety when mixed with other medications need to be cleared up!

There have been multiple marijuana-based prescription drugs available for some time including Marinol or Syndros (Dronabinol—a synthetic form of THC), which may reduce nausea/vomiting from chemotherapy and anorexia in AIDS patients. There is also Cesamet (Nabilone) and a newer CBD prescription drug known as Epidolex, as well as others cropping up in the marketplace today. All these drugs are basically synthetic cannabis-related cannabinoids, except Epidiolex, which is a plant-based pharmaceutical grade CBD extract. These products can be costly and their impact in cancer is not yet known in terms of what side effects they could reduce, or if they have any true anti-cancer properties. The other issue is the OTC versions of CBD, which in some cases have quality control (QC) and pricing issues (mentioned earlier). Always ask for a COA (certificate of analysis) when purchasing CBD, which lists the ingredients and demonstrates some QC.

There is also the issue of drug interactions because many of these products are heavily metabolized in the liver and could interact negatively with some prostate cancer pills. We just don't know at this time which drugs cause interactions because there have not been enough safety studies done in prostate cancer. The risk of DILI is there until proven otherwise. There is also the issue of dependence or even withdrawal from marijuana use, and perhaps even CBD, because the drug concentrations are higher today than ever, which theoretically increases the risk of dependence or addiction. I know, I sound like my parents when I was a kid! While CBD and other cannabinoids will have a role in medicine, and already do in some areas (e.g., rare forms of pediatric epilepsy), when it comes to many cancer issues we are unfortunately still in the early stages of understanding what it can and cannot do. A less appreciated concern with marijuana in prostate cancer is the potential for an appetite increase, which for some men on ADT, for example, is problematic because they're already at an increased risk of weight/waist gain. The bottom line is CBD and marijuana have a role in some cancer patients, and in others not so much.

Cholesterol lowering drugs (statins, PCSK9 inhibitors, etc.), but what about CoQ10? Less could mean more money saved and fewer pills after you explore all the options.

This topic was well-covered in chapter two, so please review that information to see why cholesterol lowering drugs are getting so much attention right now! The only other question when taking a statin is whether it's also appropriate to take a coenzyme Q10 (CoQ10) supplement to reduce the risk of muscle aches and pains. Maybe not and rarely maybe?! The rate of muscle and joint problems is already low with statins, so only a small percentage of people experience it. Also, taking a supplement immediately when starting a statin is like spending a bunch of money on something without evidence of whether you truly needed to spend that money in the first place. In addition, adding more pills to potentially prevent the side effect from another pill can create "pill fatigue."

Now, if you take a statin and think you're experiencing this problem then your healthcare team needs to know and test for it to determine if it's caused by the drug or another source. Ideally, you want to take a pill or injection that does not create this side effect (see Appendix 2). There are so many options today that even if you're experiencing this problem from one statin, you can generally be moved to a different statin product and/or dosage, which can give you the same cholesterol lowering result, but without the side effect. In the rare case where every option has been exhausted, and it comes down to remaining on your cholesterol lowering medication, or not, then CoQ10 could be one alternative. Again, please keep in mind that muscle problems, when they occur, happen for a variety of reasons, and not just because CoQ10 levels in the blood drop with statin drugs, which is part of the reason some studies have not found this option to be a solution to the problem while other studies have found some benefit. Finally, what is the impact of large dosages of CoQ10 supplements in prostate cancer patients? We don't know because it has not been adequately studied.

Eye Health Supplement for Age-Related Macular Degeneration (AMD) from AREDS1 and AREDS2 clinical trials for intermediate-to-advanced stages of AMD.

If your eye health medical team recommends one of the most common supplements studied to help with AMD (from the AREDS1 and AREDS2 clinical trials) first keep in mind what the National Eye Institute (NEI – part of the NIH) recommends. They suggest the following daily combination of vitamins and minerals, which can be found in products like PreserVision supplements and others, if you have at least intermediate AMD in one or both eyes, and you're trying to prevent it from becoming more advanced. Even if you have advanced AMD, this combination can be an option:

- Vitamin C-500 mg
- Vitamin E-400 IU
- Zinc-80 mg
- Copper (cupric oxide)-2 mg
- Lutein-10 mg
- Zeaxanthin-2 mg

(**Note:** *Copper was used to prevent zinc-related copper deficiency*)

This is the good news! The bad news is this combination supplement has not been shown to help with earlier stages of AMD, or to prevent AMD in people without this condition. Additionally, even though this specific formula has been shown to be the safest, it's not found in many products. First make sure you qualify and then find the right low-cost quality-controlled product.

Also, the amount of vitamin E indicated above is the same as the dosage found in the SELECT trial which was found to increase the risk of prostate cancer, so this must be a discussed with your healthcare team. Finally, older versions of this eye formula may contain beta-carotene (15 mg/day), which in supplemental form could increase the risk of lung cancer in former and current smokers. The newer versions have dropped the beta-carotene and you should too (just to be safe). Again, even if your healthcare team approves the use of this supplement then getting the safest combination tested thus far (listed above) is the way to go! It should also be kept in mind that most of the participants in the AREDS1 and AREDS2 studies also took a separate multivitamin.

Fad Diets

How can you be sure that a fad diet claiming to fight prostate cancer might be worth considering? Before you sign on for a ketogenic or high-fat diet, or a vegan diet, or a high-protein diet, or go "Paleo," consider what impact the diet will have on five key areas: (1) body mass index (BMI)/belly; (2) blood cholesterol; (3) blood pressure; (4) blood sugar; and (5) brain health (mood or mental health). If your diet is moving all the Moyad "5 B's" in a positive direction, then your medical team could support it as being heart healthy.

Fish Oil (EPA, or EPA + DHA) vs Fish?
Everything comes with a catch (pun intended)!

Fish oil comes in supplemental and prescription forms, but the prescription forms are FDA approved to lower high levels of triglycerides and can also be combined with many other cardiovascular drugs. However, fish oil has a controversial recent history where some major cardiovascular trials have not found it works better than a placebo (for example, the STRENGTH trial). While other trials demonstrated some benefit, they were tested against a controversial placebo product (i.e., mineral oil in the REDUCE-IT trial). Keep in mind that higher dosages of fish oil can increase the risk of blood thinning, and if the product contains both EPA and DHA omega-3 then at higher dosages it could also increase LDL cholesterol (prescription EPA alone has not caused regular increases in LDL). Some of the most promising research on fish oil occurred in the VITAL trial where 1000 mg/day of a prescription fish oil product (Omacor) appeared to play some role (as did vitamin D) in reducing the risk of autoimmune diseases. However, it had no impact on cancer or cardiovascular disease prevention at this more moderate dosage, and higher dosages can come with more risks. On the other hand, eating healthy sources of omega-3 fatty acids from plants or fish has demonstrated heart healthy benefits, and some anti-cancer properties.

Folic acid, the synthetic form of Folate, and the ongoing debate in prostate cancer needs to be appreciated.

First folate (vitamin B9) describes all the different forms of vitamin B9 out there including the stuff found in the diet. Folic acid is the synthetic form of folate, which has been PROVEN to reduce the risk of neural tube effects (NTDs) when women take them before and during pregnancy. This is not an issue and should be supported! The issue is whether some cancer patients, including men with prostate cancer, should be exposed to excessive amounts of folic acid outside of the diet, for example from supplements. Some physicians use folic acid and other forms of folate when they give a prescription drug that can profoundly suppress the absorption or utilization of this vitamin and increase the risk of side effects from the drug itself. For example, methotrexate which is used for some autoimmune conditions.

However, since folic acid is fortified in many products and is so easy to get from dietary sources, one could argue that most men, especially those with prostate cancer do not need to be exposed to higher amounts. There is preliminary data to suggest some cancers like to use excessive amounts of folic acid for growth (e.g., preliminary data in bladder cancer). There is also some recent, but preliminary data in prostate cancer, but since this research has not been tested in major studies what do you do? It's safe to assume getting folate from food is more than adequate/safe, and the only men with prostate cancer that need individual folic acid (folate) supplements or prescription forms are those whose healthcare teams recommend more because of their unique situation (folate reducing drugs, etc).

Should men with prostate cancer request a folate blood test occasionally along with their other tests? This is not known and although it may be an interesting result to see there is no good research to support what the ideal blood number should be in men with prostate cancer. What makes more sense is to reduce the unnecessary exposure to supplemental folic acid until more is known, and this is simply a good piece of advice when it comes to other nutritional compounds of concern (e.g., selenium, vitamin E, zinc, etc.). It's always interesting to me how the dietary sources are never the issue, but rather excessive amounts from other sources when not needed, especially when we're talking about prostate cancer.

Last, but not least, before getting any PET-CT imaging, for example PSMA PET/CT, please tell your healthcare team whether you are taking supplemental folic acid (or another form) because it has not been well-studied whether it could create a false positive result on the screen (see PSMA IMAGING chapter in other PW books). Additionally, unmetabolized folic acid (UMFA) appears to increase as we age, which again suggests most men are getting more than enough folic acid or folate from food sources.

Hyperbaric Oxygen Therapy (HBOT)

This is not an alternative medicine strictly speaking, but it deserves more attention, so it was placed in this section. Many medical centers are now offering this therapy to treat a side effect of radiation known as "radiation cystitis (RC)." RC literally means inflammation of the bladder, and though it's a fairly uncommon (5-10% of patients) side effect of radiation therapy to the pelvic area, it still occurs often enough to be a concern. RC refers to a group of potential symptoms including some or all of the following:

- Blood in the urine (hematuria)
- Frequency
- Urgency
- Pelvic Pain

RC may occur early, or in the first few weeks after radiation treatment or long after (decades later), but the average time to occurrence is approximately three years. There are many options for treating this condition, but arguably the one that receives the least amount of attention is known as "Hyperbaric Oxygen Therapy" or HBOT. If you're dealing with this or another related side effect of radiation therapy (for example non-healing radiation proctitis) then ask your healthcare team if you qualify for HBOT. The good news is that many insurance companies now cover it and although it may take 20 or more sessions to get results it may still be worth it for some patients with tough to treat issues. Also, please be sure to review the latest side effects with this therapy because research is learning more about them and although not common, they should be known before receiving this therapy (e.g., temporary visual changes, temporary ear issues, seizure risk in rare cases, etc.).

Kidney Stones and supplements—the list is unfortunately growing, but how about some amazing kidney stone prevention tips...sans pills!

Several different supplements in higher dosages have been associated with an increased risk of kidney stones including calcium (especially calcium carbonate), inosine, vitamin C, vitamin D, and potentially many others. It's another reason to adhere to "more is not better" when it comes to many things. With that in mind, the following table lists some of the best lifestyle tips to prevent kidney stones!

My Top 11 List for Preventing Kidney Stones
1. Increase your intake of dietary potassium, which naturally increases your intake of dietary calcium, fiber and magnesium and lowers your intake of sodium, which collectively lowers your risk of kidney stones (and as a bonus appears to lower the risk of osteoporosis).*
2. Drink enough fluid daily to be hydrated or have clear colored urine.
3. Maintain a healthy waist/weight, which helps keep the urine healthy.
4. Exercise regularly (yes, this also reduces stone risk).
5. Don't mega-dose on supplements that can increase oxalate, like vitamin C.

6. Don't take calcium supplements for bone health until you try to first get it from dietary sources since it's so easy to get calcium from foods. A normal intake of dietary calcium (1,000–1,200 mg per day based on age and male/female) is associated with a reduced risk of kidney stones (too little or too much can cause stones). You were not meant to always take pills! If you take a thiazide (and possibly potassium sparing) diuretic pill than keep in mind it can already increase the amount of calcium in your blood (body), so be careful and do not immediately take extra calcium (or vitamin D). On the other hand, "loop diuretics" can increase calcium loss in urine, prednisone can reduce calcium absorption, and when taking ADT you want to be sure to get the recommended amounts of calcium and vitamin D, so ask your healthcare team how your medications may impact calcium in your body.

7. Do not mega-dose or take vitamin D supplements unless really needed because this can increase the amount of calcium in your blood and urine and increase the risk of calcium stones

8. Consume less sodium to prevent calcium from spilling into your urine in large amounts.

9. Reduce or moderate animal (non-dairy) protein intake (especially if this is causing the 5 B's to become abnormal). Animal protein (meats) also can increase the amount of uric acid in the urine (another risk factor for stones). Protein from fish and plant sources do not appear to increase the risk of kidney stones and have many other ingredients that are kidney healthy.

10. Quit smoking or using any tobacco (including secondhand exposure). Smoking appears to increase the risk of kidney stones, according to some preliminary research.

11. Stay heart healthy = kidney healthy = stone prevention (gee, what a shocker)!

Note: *The DASH diet (high in dietary potassium, magnesium, fiber, etc., and low in sodium, sugar, etc.) discussed in Appendix 3 with blood pressure (and the diet chapter) continues to accumulate wonderful research suggesting it reduces the risk of kidney stones while simultaneously lowering blood pressure.*

L-citrulline, L-arginine and other ED supplements are getting some positive attention.

There is renewed interest and positive data in using these supplements along with conventional medicine for penile rehabilitation before, during and after prostate cancer treatment. L-citrulline may work similarly to L-arginine, but at half the dosage. Both supplements have an ability to reduce blood pressure and have not been tested adequately in patients with existing cardiovascular disease (CVD), so talk to your healthcare team about the latest safety, dosage, and efficacy data. Korean Red Ginseng (a form of Panax ginseng), and even MACA (Peru-based or derived) has preliminary evidence it may help some men with ED, but again this is preliminary, and as stated at the beginning of this chapter, "herbals are a different animal."

Lycopene—you say tomato and I say "asparagus"?!

Lycopene supplements have not received enough research to determine if they should be used with prostate cancer treatment, and most of the positive data comes from food sources of lycopene. This is another reason to improve the quality of your diet, and not to necessarily focus on the tomato (one of the largest sources of lycopene) unless you love tomatoes. Here is surprising research: Asparagus was also found to have a small amount of lycopene! Yes! So, one could theoretically argue asparagus is one of the better sources of lycopene (and odorous urine – sorry had to add that for fun) per calorie compared to many other moderate or higher caloric sources. Regardless, eating healthier means you increase your healthy dietary patterns and not focus on one food because of a single ingredient found in that food, unless again, you just love tomatoes (like me, but I also love asparagus). Other foods with lycopene include apricots, guava, papaya, pink grapefruit, watermelon, and more. Thus, originally, the positive research on lycopene suggested the solution was to eat more fruits and vegetables daily, but somehow this message got lost over the years, and hopefully we can get back to that today!

Melatonin—you can make it, or take it, but making it makes more "cents!"

Melatonin supplements in excess can cause next day fatigue/drowsiness and blood pressure drug interference. Melatonin supplements at lower dosages than commonly advertised (1-3 mg) could be helpful if you are having trouble sleeping, and your healthcare team approves. Melatonin is sold in different forms and is commonly used as a prescription drug in Europe and many other countries around the world. For example, it can be prescribed as a 2 mg prolonged release (PR) tablet (such as "Circadin") throughout Europe. In the U.S. there are a few prescriptions that help with sleep that impact the melatonin receptors (for example "ramelteon"), and the potential side effects from these prescriptions should also be similarly applied to melatonin supplements until proven otherwise. For example, do not take it with the drug fluvoxamine (it can increase toxicity), or high-fat meals (delays the absorption). Also, higher/mega-dosages of melatonin could reduce testosterone and increase prolactin.

OTC melatonin is popular, but to ensure that what you're buying is really what you're getting be sure to look for a quality control (QC) symbol. Past research has shown some QC problems with some OTC products. There are also concerns over combining melatonin with any other type of sleep medications or alcohol, and again when individuals take higher dosages of melatonin it can increase the risk of toxicity. Although one of the most studied dosages is approximately 2-3 mg/day (the physiologic dose or what the body makes for sleep is often less than 1 mg), for some reason these lower dosages do not receive enough attention. Melatonin should only be taken occasionally as needed, and not every day. It's also used for jet lag and in people with REM sleep behavior disorder. Beta-blocker drugs have been shown to lower melatonin levels in the body.

Regardless, with all the talk and excitement for melatonin pills, what tends to get overshadowed is your own levels of body melatonin can increase if you follow proper sleep hygiene (see the 5 BBs chapter for some wonderful tips). For example, reducing or eliminating any light in the bedroom when sleeping, and minimizing exposure from computers or cell phones several hours before bed can boost melatonin. Increasing your own body levels of melatonin, before trying the pills, should have its own TV commercial or advertisement. Unfortunately, this book may be the only place you'll always see this advertised!

Multivitamin(s) and male physicians provide lessons?! Yes! But, what about the newly discovered COSMOS?! One or half of one is plenty (when one is needed), and in many other cases none! The only multivitamin tested in a rigorous phase 3 type trial included over 14,000 men for a little more than 11 years and was known as "PHS2" (Physicians' Health Study 2). The product they used was Centrum Silver (one per day) versus a placebo. The multivitamin appeared to be associated with no impact on prostate cancer risk but did show a slight reduction in the risk of cancer in general (also eye cataracts). This is not an endorsement of Centrum Silver, but rather transparency, or consumers knowing what product was used in the most rigorous randomized trial (just as we demand to know with prescription medications), and thus having some standard to compare to when purchasing any multivitamin. If you decide to take a multivitamin, it's important to read labels and be aware of the ingredients and amounts of vitamins and minerals, as well as how "clean" the product is in terms of QC.

While multivitamins can be beneficial, there is some evidence that suggests taking more than one multivitamin a day has no incremental benefit and could even encourage prostate cancer growth from some well-done observational studies (NIH-AARP Diet & Health Study, etc.), so this should be avoided in prostate cancer patients (better to be safe). Another issue to consider is the increasing list of ingredients and amounts in multivitamins, which means it's an ever moving and larger target. So before taking any multivitamin, please talk to your healthcare team to determine if there is a reason to take one, and if so, which one they recommend. Some healthcare teams like the fact that B12, extra calcium, vitamin D and other nutrients can all be found in one pill, but the reality is the amount of selenium, vitamin E, and other nutrients in any multivitamin product should be discussed. In the past, a multivitamin was truly one pill, but today it could be many pills, depending on the company's definition. Some companies are moving toward "mini" multivitamins where you take two small pills a day which equates to one regular pill. However, there is nothing stopping you from taking just one mini pill a day or every few days, or a children's multivitamin, if your healthcare team thinks that is more than fine (because the lower dosage is often enough).

Regardless, do you even need a multivitamin today? The most recent phase 3 trial (randomized, double-blind, and placebo-controlled) conducted to try and answer this question was released. It's known as "COSMOS," and once again a daily Centrum Silver was used versus a placebo. There were over 21,000 participants, but this time it included women and men, and although the median follow-up was very short (only 3.6 years) it had not reduced the risk of invasive cancer (including prostate cancer), even in those with a history of cancer, and it did not reduce the risk of cardiovascular disease (CVD). This would suggest that generally healthy individuals with a moderately healthy diet or lifestyle may not need a multivitamin. However, COSMOS will have multiple updates in the future, and as explained earlier, some people may need to take a multivitamin to normalize a deficiency or insufficiency when they are unable to fix the problem via diet alone (for example B12, calcium, vitamin D, etc.). Otherwise, many people could argue today that the modest benefits, or no effect in general, from phase 3 trials of men and women are not impressive enough to take a daily multivitamin. Still, you don't have to look through a telescope at night to get COSMOS updates, but rather ask your healthcare team about the latest and greatest information. (Sorry, but that was the best pun I could create in the moment.)

Probiotics and the microbiome are amazing especially if you can change your biome via lifestyle changes!

When it comes to prostate cancer, probiotics simply do not have evidence, either good or bad, as to whether they can make a side effect of treatment better, worse, or do nothing. It simply has not reached prime time yet in this area. I think what should reach prime time is the new research suggesting that every time someone makes a heart healthy change, the microbiome (the microbes that naturally live in our bodies and produce vitamins, boost immunity, and protect us from germs) becomes healthier and more diverse in response to that wonderful change. Where the heck is that commercial? Eating better, losing weight, exercising and all the other stuff this book preaches can improve your microbiome! Recent preliminary research also suggests DIETARY fiber improves your microbiome and may improve the response to some preventive vaccines and immune therapies for cancer, but this human research is again, preliminary at best. Even if it turns out to be incorrect, there are still countless reasons to improve your dietary fiber intake (again, it keeps your intestinal train running on time)!

Quercetin for chronic non-bacterial prostatitis

Chronic non-bacterial prostatitis/chronic pelvic pain syndrome (CP/CPPS) is a common condition in men that causes pain and inflammation in the prostate, pelvis, and urinary tract. The good news is quercetin and other supplements (cernilton, etc.) have some positive preliminary clinical data that shows it can treat some forms of CP/CPPS (along with conventional treatment). However, in prostate cancer, there is not enough research to suggest it provides a benefit or causes harm. Vegetables and fruits are good sources of quercetin, and isn't that interesting?

Selenium and/or Vitamin E as individual supplements were not what prostate cancer researchers thought they would be, and it served to be one of the greatest lessons in prostate and many other cancers.

Selenium supplements, in general, have not been shown to be beneficial against prostate cancer. In fact, some studies have suggested they could increase the risk of prostate cancer progression, especially in men with adequate or high intakes of selenium from diet who also take a separate selenium supplement. Selenium from food or even in some one per day multivitamins have not been the major concern, but rather the individual 200 microgram (or more) supplements, or higher, which have been preliminarily concerning in prostate cancer patients.

Vitamin E was already well covered earlier in this chapter, and unless you're already taking it in lower dosages in a multivitamin, or because it's a part of your macular degeneration product, then it's best to avoid individual vitamin E supplements, especially at the dosage used in the SELECT trial (400 IU). The SELECT trial was one the first phase 3 type supplement clinical trials in medical history to demonstrate that when it comes to prostate cancer prevention, more is not always better in otherwise healthy men. It was a groundbreaking finding, which changed the landscape of prostate cancer in many ways because up until this time there was a plethora of indirect (laboratory and observational data, etc.) information suggesting more vitamin E could be better. This is the essence of evidence-based medicine. If you're dealing with prostate cancer than try to avoid individual selenium and vitamin E supplements (single multivitamin is usually okay) because of where the evidence is today! It's also interesting how many healthy food sources (e.g., salmon, garlic, nuts, oatmeal, seeds, whole wheat pasta, etc.) contain plenty of selenium and even vitamin E in many cases, which suggests food sources are the way to go (as usual)!

Tea and Tea-derived supplements—stick with the tea for two!

Most forms of tea, including black, green, herbal, oolong, etc. are healthy and have few or no calories. There is also plenty of research to demonstrate they are heart healthy. Additionally, drinking tea is associated with other healthy behaviors, which is why taking tea-based supplements may seem interesting, but currently the evidence supports drinking tea versus taking supplements. Keep in mind, if you're on the blood thinner warfarin than green tea, which could contain a large amount of vitamin K, may not be advisable. Please check those labels.

Weight Loss Drugs such as "Semaglutide or "Tirzepatide" could be a potential game changers?

Arguably, the generic drug known as "metformin" may be one of the best and safest medications used to prevent type 2 diabetes. Metformin is also being studied to reduce side effects from ADT. Additionally, it helps with a moderate amount of weight loss. The problem with other weight loss medications in the past is they were, paradoxically, not heart healthy. Metformin looks interesting to prevent diabetes and other metabolic issues in prostate cancer, and although it's garnering some positive research as an anti-cancer drug, it currently has more research to prevent side effects than to prevent prostate cancer progression (but more will be known soon).

Recently, a diabetes drug known as "semaglutide" appears to not only be associated with outstanding weight loss in some folks, but it has been generally safe thus far after being studied for several years. The problem with this drug could be cost, insurance coverage and the need for long-term use, but you can talk to your healthcare team. Semaglutide is a glucagon-like peptide (GLP-1), which is a hormone normally secreted by the gut that helps to regulate appetite. It's important to realize this drug helps someone eat less and therefore consume less calories, which is also what bariatric surgery does. So, when the drug is stopped then many people could gain some or most of the weight back, which again means long-term use of this product is the rule and not the exception. Also, since the drug has not been out for a long time one has to expect some side effect surprises over time (e.g., gallbladder issues). Nausea and an aversion to food is also not uncommon, which is why hearing about the latest pros and cons from your healthcare team is even more critical here. Regardless, currently semaglutide or tirezepatide look promising and are worthy of a discussion with your healthcare team if you need to lose weight. The other medications and weight loss products out there are not as exciting. Of course, when it comes to weight loss everyone is trying to find the magic pill, so asking your healthcare team about the latest, greatest, and not so great products should occur on a regular basis.

Zinc supplements in excess = not good, but they have a role in other situations.

High dosages of zinc supplements (100 mg or more) taken over many years have been associated with an increased risk of prostate problems. In addition, zinc, and other supplements (i.e., calcium, iron, magnesium, and selenium) could reduce the efficacy of the proven anti-viral influenza drug baloxavir marboxil (Xolfuza), so you don't want to take these things when on this drug. Zinc in the eye formula mentioned earlier (80 mg), or at lower dosages (in a multivitamin for example) used to reduce cold symptoms or the duration of a cold appears safe, but it can upset the stomach and cause nausea when taking individual supplements for too long. Everything comes with a catch (like fish oil)! It's also critical to keep in mind if you take individual zinc supplements daily, or regularly, you could develop low levels of copper, which in some cases can cause a rare form of anemia. So, zinc for prostate health is over hyped, especially at the larger dosages, but it may have a role as a part of the eye health formula mentioned in this chapter, or in temporary use against cold and flu symptoms (but not when taking the flu drug known as "Xofluza").

ZERO = your heart disease risk.

While practically it is impossible to reduce any risk to zero, you should pursue lifestyle changes and take supplements that have proven to be heart healthy because these are the ones most likely to have an anti–prostate cancer effect. Additionally, "zero" should represent your tolerance for taking any pill without completely analyzing whether the benefit outweighs the risk. Most AdvPCa patients should avoid taking any supplements unless there is a specific side effect or condition that requires it. Always consult with your medical team before adding any new supplement or over-the-counter medication to your treatment regime.

As we reach the end of this book, we hope that we've been successful in presenting you with a wealth of information on treatment options for AdvPCa and useful tips for managing your treatment side effects. The content here is meant to provide a basis for continuing discussions with your medical team to determine the best course of action for your individual situation. As noted, research continues all the time, and new treatment options regularly become available, so it is always important to continue to expand your knowledge about the disease. Always remember, knowledge and action equal power in dealing with your cancer. Please turn to the Appendix for more information on being heart healthy because Heart Healthy = Prostate Healthy = Head-to-Toe Healthier!

PW Lifestyle Empowerment Moment

Fast A-to-Z Pill Reduction Advice to Discuss with your Healthcare Team

("Find health in places where you did not know it existed")

Healthy weight loss reduces inflammation and can increase the blood level of many nutrients, because less inflammation allows the body to function more efficiently. Even if you need to take a supplement for some nutrient that you simply cannot get from diet or weight loss, then it's possible to get the amount you need from a children's or low dose multivitamin once a day, or even just once or twice a week in some cases (for example, B12, calcium, vitamin D, etc.). Otherwise, for most people there are plenty of non-pill options. Remember, less is more!

Thinking of Pill in terms of _____?	First how about these non-pill options?*
B12	B12 fortified foods including some plant-based milks, or high in omega-3 protein and other nutrient fish (salmon, etc.).
Calcium and/or vitamin D (Note: See calcium food sources table in this chapter.)	Most, or all can now come from the diet because of the fortification of plant-based milks and other food sources. Also, losing weight can increase vitamin D blood levels.
Fiber-based pills and powders	Fiber from dietary sources is awesome and easy to get today. In clinical studies, chia seed, flax seed powders, oatmeal, kiwis, and countless other sources (veggies, fruits, beans, lentils, beans, whole grains, etc.) have research to suggest they could work just as well as some of those pills and powders.
Fish Oil	Fish have multiple healthy nutrients (vitamin D, protein, etc.) and not just Omega-3. If you don't like fish then eat plants, because they are loaded with another type of omega-3 (ALA) that can be converted in small amounts to some fish type omega-3s (EPA) in the body.
Folic Acid (vitamin B9)	Few men with prostate cancer need more than what they get from fortified food sources. If you need more proof, then have your healthcare team check your blood level.
Green Tea	The drink contains a moderate amount of caffeine along with a stress relieving amino acid known as L-theanine and other nutrients. At zero calories, lower cost, and the flexibility of being served hot or cold, they are the winner over the pills.

Lycopene	Healthy food sources (asparagus, tomatoes, etc.) are the way to go, and has most of the positive evidence. They are also heart healthy.
Magnesium, potassium and...	Whole plant-based foods contain numerous diverse healthy nutrients, including calcium, magnesium, potassium, fiber, and more, and tend to contain minimal-to-no unhealthy nutrients (low or no cholesterol, sodium, sugar, unhealthy fats, etc.).
Mushrooms	Diverse healthy nutrients include potassium, and even vitamin D in some cases. Pill sources used against cancer have mixed data, so why not go with the food source?!
Probiotics	Heart healthy lifestyles create healthier microbiomes or healthier gut health! Where is that commercial?
Quercetin	If it really reduces inflammation, then a variety of plant-based foods (especially veggies and fruits) are tremendous sources of this compound, as well as being heart healthy.
Selenium and vitamin E	Healthy food sources have most of the cancer prevention or anti-cancer research, and not the pills (especially when it comes to prostate cancer—these pills should be avoided/discouraged for prostate cancer).
Soy	Traditional soy sources (edamame, soy milk, tempeh, tofu, etc.) dominate the positive heart healthy research and provide a wonderful source of plant protein. Soy sauce? Not so much (sorry), but who doesn't love it with sushi? Choose the low-sodium option please.

Vitamin C	Excessive amounts of vitamin C supplements can increase oxalate and kidney stones, whereas plant sources of vitamin C are kidney friendly and heart healthy!
Zinc	The RDA for zinc is approximately 8-11 mg only, which can be easily achieved from a moderately healthy diet, which includes pumpkin and other seeds, beans, nuts, oatmeal, seafood, etc.

*Note: *Almost any other nutrient that gets some positive attention in prostate cancer has a healthy food option(s) that not only provides ample amounts of a specific nutrient, but many other heart healthy nutrients that are also associated with prostate health. Fewer pills equal more money to spend on healthy food, vacations, exercise equipment, trainer, classes of all types (cooking, dance, Pilates, qigong, tai chi, yoga, etc.)! Seriously, shifting your health spending dollars from one area to another is also about being challenged to "find health in places where you did not know it existed" (another one of my favorite teaching mantras)! "Lifestyle changes can change lives!" or "lifestyle changes change lives!" (two more of my favorites of course).*

PW Lifestyle Empowerment Moment

Do you know exactly what's in that OTC or another pill?

Eating or living cleaner should be an educational, fun, interesting, and subtle process, but many people in my experience tend to apply this criterion to adult and baby food, cleaning products, or many other things besides their pills. I think this is simply an awareness issue. Some over the counter (OTC) products (including pills and fly-by-night products) could contain any of the following A-to-Z list of ingredients below, which is why this chapter started with QC and must end on QC!

This is not to imply that all these ingredients are bad. Some could be fine, but when taking a pill then the quality and quantity (QQ) of these and other ingredients would be nice to know, along with the latest safety information (just knowing the active ingredient is not enough in many cases today). Again, outstanding QC by any company is important to me because I think it further elevates the reputation of supplements, which is what I want to see because many supplements have a wonderful place in medicine (when specifically needed, like any pill). Unfortunately, it's the small percentage of bad players that appear to garner the attention, which can then get embellished by those not familiar with all those good supplement companies out there. Anyhow, here is that partial A-to-Z list!

- Additives
- Allergens
- Aluminum
- Animal products
- Anti-caking ingredients (stop ingredients from clogging up machines)
- Arsenic
- Artificial colors, flavors, ingredients, or sweeteners

- Bacteria, yeast, or mold
- Binders (make sure ingredients stick together in pills)
- Bulking agents (fill the content of pills)
- Cadmium
- Coatings (makes swallowing easier)
- Container not always biodegradable or with bisphenol-A
- Dyes (coloring) of all kinds (blue#1, #2, green #3, red #3, #40, yellow #5, #6, etc. "hike!"—pun intended)
- Fillers (add more volume to pills—could even be hydrogenated oils)
- Fluoride
- Fragrances
- Gluten
- GMO (controversial)
- Herbicides/Pesticides
- Hormones
- Lead
- Lubricants (prevent pills from sticking to manufacturing equipment)
- Mercury
- MSG
- PCBs
- Pesticide residues
- Preservatives
- Sodium
- Silicon dioxide
- Sugar alcohols
- Sugar in many forms) dextrose, glucose, lactose, etc.)
- Titanium dioxide
- Etc. Etc. Etc.

Please always talk to your medical team.

Appendix—

Bonus Material

Appendix—Bonus Material

Heart Healthy = Prostate Healthy = Head-to-Toe Healthier
Heart Healthy Numbers & Behaviors

Did you know that becoming heart healthy may be the most important thing you can do when facing prostate cancer and improving your overall health? Over the last 30 years there has been a consistent emphasis from clinical studies to become more heart healthy regardless of your prostate cancer situation (i.e., at risk, diagnosed, treated for localized cancer, locally advanced cancer, or advanced prostate cancer). Improving the numbers related to heart health such as your weight (including BMI and waist circumference), blood cholesterol, blood pressure, and blood sugar through lifestyle (behavioral) and medications, when needed, has been linked to disease prevention and recovery, along with better quality of life and longevity. Here are some surprising findings from studies that have stood the true test of time!

- The number one cause of death in men and women is cardiovascular disease (CVD), and this has been the case for over 100 consecutive years!

- The number one cause of death in men diagnosed with prostate cancer is still CVD because it is such a massive and common (high probability) problem throughout life. Most men with prostate cancer are already at a high risk for a cardiovascular disease at the time of diagnosis. And, if prostate cancer becomes more advanced then the cancer itself can raise the risk of a cardiovascular problem by increasing the amount of inflammation in the body. In addition, some very effective treatments for prostate cancer can potentially and paradoxically increase the risk of cardiovascular problems by causing weight gain, high blood cholesterol, high blood pressure, and/or high blood sugar in some patients.

- Unhealthy behaviors (lifestyle) and heart health indicators could potentially increase the risk of being diagnosed with a more aggressive prostate cancer, or even increase the risk of prostate cancer recurrence (returning) after treatment.

But Here Comes the Amazing News...

- Heart healthy numbers and behaviors could potentially reduce the risk of being diagnosed with more lethal prostate cancer, or even reduce the risk in some men that are at a higher genetic/family risk of potentially developing more aggressive prostate cancer. Just because you were given a bad set of genes doesn't always mean you were destined to wear those bad genes your entire life. Healthy numbers and behaviors could reduce the risk of those genes being expressed or activated, as well as contributing to overall health.

- Heart healthy numbers and behaviors could potentially reduce the risk of prostate cancer recurrence after treatment, death from prostate cancer, and even side effects of many prostate cancer treatments, where in some cases paradoxically these very effective cancer medications or conventional treatments can increase some aspect of our CVD risk. Therefore, heart healthy numbers and behaviors could potentially help reduce some of the side effects of many prostate cancer treatments today!

- Heart healthy behaviors and numbers could potentially reduce the risk and severity of other common prostate issues such as BPH (benign prostatic hyperplasia) or non-cancerous prostate enlargement, which can increase the risk of kidney, sexual, and urinary problems, as well as cause increases in your PSA.

- Heart healthy behaviors and numbers could potentially reduce the risk of some types of chronic prostate inflammation (prostatitis) and sexual dysfunction.

- Heart healthy behaviors and numbers could potentially increase the chances a man or woman lives better and longer than at any other time during history! If you look at the research of the longest-lived populations in the world with some of the highest levels of quality of life, they all have something in common: They are some of the heart healthiest places on earth! They have been historically known as "Blue Zones," but I also like to think of them as "heart healthy first and foremost zones!"

The bottom line: Whatever turns out to be healthy for the heart is healthy for the entire body, from our heads (the brain) to our toes. The best way to prevent the most common causes of health problems and reduced longevity as we age is to try and achieve optimal heart health. It's the common path that leads to and from all the different parts of the body, maximizing your overall mental and physical health.

For example, quitting smoking does not just reduce the risk of many cancers, or cancer returning after treatment, but also reduces the risk of hearing loss, erectile dysfunction, and cardiovascular events (i.e., heart attacks, strokes, etc.). Similarly, other healthy lifestyle changes can positively impact your head-to-toe health (more on this later). The bad news is cardiovascular disease continues to be the number one cause of mortality; but the good is news is that over the last 100+ years research continues to demonstrate that heart healthy behaviors and numbers are associated with an increased chance of a healthier body and mind!

What Can a Healthy Heart Do for You?

The following table illustrates why nothing can beat the awesome power of being heart healthy in terms of overall health advice.

Heart Healthy = Head-to-Toe Healthy	The Potential Impact of Achieving Optimal Heart Health
Artery (and all types of blood vessels) healthy	Reduces risk of weakness (aneurysms) and tears/rips (dissection) of arteries that can be life threatening, and reduces the risk of blockages in large, medium, and small arteries and other blood vessels that carry blood, oxygen, nutrients, and waste from every part of the body. (Blockage in the carotid artery, for example, can lead to debilitating stroke, blindness and more.)
Bladder healthy	Reduces risk of bladder cancer and bladder conditions, such as incontinence and OAB (overactive bladder).
Bone and balance healthy	Reduces risk of bone loss, osteoporosis, falls, and life-threatening bone fractures, which often require long-term nursing home care.
Brain healthy	Reduces risk of memory issues, Alzheimer's/dementia and Parkinson's disease severity (cognitive issues), per some preliminary new research.
Breast healthy	Reduces risk of aggressive breast cancer.
Colon healthy	Reduces risk of aggressive colon cancer and experiencing colon-related problems, such as polyps, hemorrhoids, and constipation.

DNA healthy	Reduces risk of expressing a mutated gene that can cause harm or death, and/or delays the appearance of a mutated or spontaneous unhealthy genetic change.
Ear healthy	Reduces risk of hearing loss.
Eye healthy	Reduces risk of major eye diseases that can cause vision loss (AMD, cataracts, diabetic retinopathy, glaucoma and more).
Family Anti-Disease healthy	Men, along with their partners and families, often want to know the best advice for their sons or daughters on reducing the risk of future aggressive cancers, including prostate cancer. Thus far, the best evidence apart from being more closely monitored and potentially genetically tested as adults (if they qualify) is tell your kids to reduce their risk of cardiovascular disease to as close to ZERO as possible. This appears to help discourage lethal or aggressive prostate cancer genes or other factors from being activated. It also increases their chances of improved quality of life and longevity. Pay it forward please!
Hormone (adrenal) healthy	Reduces the risk of abnormal hormone production from various organs, including the adrenal glands. It even helps to reduce stress hormone levels such as cortisol. Hormone changes from weight gain alone increase the risk of some cancers and medical conditions (such as PCOS and low testosterone). These unhealthy hormone changes are now increasing in obese children as well as adults.

Immune system healthy	Reduces risk of being hospitalized for and dying from infectious diseases like the flu, pneumonia, and COVID-19. It improves immune surveillance to prevent and fight chronic diseases, such as cancer and reduces risk of some auto-immune conditions.
Inflammation healthy (aka "anti-inflammation healthy")	Reduces risk of inflammatory diseases, such as gout, and of acute inflammation turning into chronic inflammation that can damage most areas of the body.
Joint healthy	Reduces risk of experiencing severe pain from osteoarthritis and the need for invasive procedures.
Kidney healthy	Reduces risk of kidney stones, kidney cancer, kidney failure, dialysis, and need for a kidney transplant.
Limb (legs, arms) healthy	Reduces risk of potentially life-threatening blood clots and circulation/nerve problems, such as peripheral artery disease (PAD), peripheral neuropathy, and other micro-circulation problems, that could result in long-term injury/consequences.
Liver healthy	Reduces risk of fatty liver, liver damage and the need for liver transplant.
Lung healthy	Reduces risk of lung cancer (#1 cancer killer) and COPD (fifth leading cause of death in women and men).

Medication healthy	Numerous medications used to control blood pressure, blood cholesterol, blood sugar, and other issues have a better chance of working well or being more effective when someone takes care of their overall heart health. It helps minimize side effects from many medications because a lower dosage is needed for effectiveness.
Mental/emotional healthy (I could have put this under brain health, but it is too important to share with another category.)	New evidence suggests a potential reduced risk of stress, anxiety, depression, and pervasive negative thinking ("catastrophizing") that could lead to so many other problems. The improvement in mental health stimulates better physical health and vice versa. Heart healthy behaviors may also further enhance the benefits of medications for these conditions.
Microbiome/ gut healthy	Increases the chances that healthy bacteria will take up residence in your gut versus nasty, mean, unhealthy bacteria.
Nerve healthy	Nerves rely on healthy blood flow for survival, including the nerves in the head, skin, eyes, penis, toes, etc.
Pancreas healthy	Reduces risk of pancreatic damage, diabetes, and pancreatic cancer.
Prostate healthy	Reduces risk of aggressive prostate cancer, recurrence, and of suffering from a severe form of non-cancerous prostate enlargement (BPH) that impacts the ability to urinate. Reduces some forms of chronic prostate inflammation.

Reproductive/ sexual organ(s) healthy	Reduces risk of infertility in women and men, and cancer of the reproductive organs.
Sexual function healthy	Reduces risk of erectile and female sexual dysfunction (ED & FSD).
Skin healthy	Reduces risk of skin damage, signs of aging, and skin ulcers and infections.
Stomach and esophagus healthy	Reduces risk of acid reflux, and stomach and esophageal cancer.
Thyroid healthy (Note: Thyroid dysfunction has also been known as a cause of heart dysfunction, so that train runs in both directions.)	Reduces risk of thyroid disease/cancer and improves thyroid function and uptake of important levels of thyroid hormone within the heart itself.
_____ healthy	Feel free to add any other parts of the human body to this list!

Now, how can you and your family achieve optimal heart, prostate, and overall head-to-toe health? Many of the answers to optimal heart health can be found in this book! We'll try to answer the most common questions, including: How do you know if your lifestyle changes and medications (if needed) are really working? How do you really know if you're becoming the heart healthiest version of you? How do you know if eating something not so healthy (occasionally) is really making you unhealthy or not? The answers to these questions and more start with the 5 Barometers or B's for Better Health! So, please turn the page and let's get started! **Lifestyle changes change lives!**

Appendix 1—The First B = Belly/BMI

Weight/Waist Healthy = Head-to-Toe Healthier

If you're carrying excess pounds or kilograms, weight or waist loss is the most important B of the bunch when it comes to head-to-toe health. Unhealthy weight gain can make some of the potential side effects of localized, locally advanced, or advanced prostate cancer treatment worse (e.g., erectile dysfunction, incontinence) regardless of the treatment you've had or are still receiving. For example, when receiving androgen deprivation treatment (ADT) weight gain can make hot flashes more severe and could increase the risk of nerve damage from chemotherapy. In addition, weight gain generally increases the risk of cancer-related fatigue (CRF), and there is enough preliminary evidence to suggest it could even increase your potential risk of cancer returning after treatment. It has been known for some time that excess weight could increase the risk of being diagnosed with aggressive cancer, but only recently has the research suggested it could also negatively impact prognosis.

Of course, this data is just preliminary right now. What if a healthy weight is never proven to reduce the risk of prostate cancer relapse/recurrence or negatively impact prognosis? Even if that were the case an unhealthy weight or waist circumference is still heart unhealthy and can reduce the quality and quantity of your life, which is why it's the first B we need to cover. If these facts are not convincing enough than keep in mind most men today (and women) are either overweight or obese, so there is an urgent need to address these issues. Furthermore, ADT paradoxically increases the risk of weight gain by reducing metabolism despite being able to fight prostate cancer. This, combined with the fact that our metabolism slows down as we age, makes it even harder to lose excess weight when dealing with some form of prostate cancer treatment. Also, as you lose weight hunger or appetite can temporarily increase and metabolism can slow down even further as your body tries harder to hold on to the excess pounds (or kilograms) it has at that moment! For some folks, there are also some genetics involved making it hard to shed weight compared to others—even within the same family! Ugh! So, again it needs to be the first B we address in this book.

The great news is that any healthy dietary program should allow you to start seeing weight loss in the first week or two. Later in this book we will help you work with your medical or healthcare team to achieve your maximum healthy weight loss with countless tips!

However, let's continue to talk about the impact that unhealthy weight gain has on a variety of conditions or different parts of the body, further demonstrating why it can make many of the side effects of prostate cancer treatment much worse. Obesity is now the primary preventable cause of illness and premature death globally; it has pushed smoking to the number two spot. According to the National Institutes of Health, more than two-thirds—70 percent—of U.S. adults are overweight or obese today. If the current trends continue, by the time the next edition of this book is released in a few years, about three out of every four—75 percent—of the population will be overweight or obese!

Added weight, especially those pounds that creep on around your middle increases chronic inflammation in your body. Some "experts" used to believe that adipose tissue (aka "fat") wasn't very metabolically active. They thought the fat cells just sat there, not doing much of anything except causing frustration. This theory turned out to be not accurate (cue the buzzer sound, folks). Fat produces and releases numerous inflammatory compounds that can increase chronic inflammation from head to toe. Adipose tissue, for example, can potentially increase numerous compounds secreted by inflammatory cells cranking up inflammation more and more. This acts like a fertilizer to not only encourage some unhealthy cells to become unhealthier, but to grow beyond their normal borders and move toward other parts of the body. Excess weight not only increases the risk of countless diseases (see the list below), but it also makes many of those same medical conditions worse and more difficult to treat. It's amazing to think that you can impact so many body systems by making one positive change—limiting weight/waist gain (aka trying to achieve a healthier weight and/or waist—though it may not be easy.

Table: A Short List of the Medical Conditions Impacted by Obesity

(by either increasing risk or increasing the risk of things getting worse (severity) or even potentially reducing the impact of conventional treatment in some cases)

Acid reflux (GERD)	**Dementia** (Alzheimer's, memory loss, etc.)
Atrial fibrillation	**Diabetes**
Blood clots	**Eye diseases that can lead to blindness**
BPH (Benign Prostatic Hyperplasia or non-cancerous enlargement of the prostate)	**Fetal defects from maternal obesity**
Breathlessness	**Gallbladder disease**
Cancer (breast, cervix, colorectal, endometrial, esophageal, gallbladder, kidney, liver, multiple myeloma, non-Hodgkin's lymphoma, ovarian, pancreas, pediatric, and prostate). Obesity may also increase the risk of having a more aggressive form of cancer.	**Gout**
Complications from surgical procedures	**Headaches (migraine)**
COVID-19 (higher risk of more severe disease and hospitalizations)	**Heart disease**

Heart failure	**Low back pain** (chronic) and other potential chronic pain syndromes
Hiatal hernia	**Low testosterone**
High blood pressure	**NAFLD/NASH** (aka fatty liver)
High cholesterol	**Osteoarthritis (OA)**
Hot flashes (more severe)	**Osteoporosis** and fracture risk at specific bone sites
Idiopathic intracranial hypertension (IIH)	**Peripheral artery disease (PAD)**
Immobility	**Peripheral neuropathy (PN)**
Incontinence	**Polycystic ovarian syndrome (PCOS)**
Infertility (men and women)	**Pregnancy complications** (preeclampsia, etc.)
Kidney diseases including kidney stones, chronic kidney disease (CKD), kidney failure, and need for dialysis	**Prostate cancer** risk, recurrence, and could compromise the effectiveness of some treatments, or at the least increase the risk of more severe side effects from treatment.

Psoriasis	**Stroke**
Psoriatic arthritis (PsA) and other inflammatory joint diseases	**Urinary tract infection**
Restless leg syndrome (RLS)	**Vaccine (adult)** responses could be compromised
Sexual dysfunction (female sexual dysfunction & erectile dysfunction)	**Varicose veins**
Sleep apnea	

PW Lifestyle Empowerment Moment

Weight drop = healthy testosterone pop (if needed)!

Many men want to increase their testosterone for a variety of reasons, and they turn to pills and injections and all kinds of other things to increase it when it's low. What gets missed is the past research on weight loss as a first option to increase your testosterone "naturally." According to numerous studies, approximately 10-15% of body weight loss has been associated with dramatic increases in testosterone for many men needing to lose weight. These results are, at times, similar to what would have occurred if they received low-dose testosterone drug therapy! However, some men may not see a large surge in testosterone with weight loss. If that's the case, then at least other heart healthy benefits are observed—and it's a wonderful way of finding out if your body will still make more testosterone with weight loss, or if you need to even entertain other options for improving this number!

Lifestyle changes are considered first-line treatment options for so many heart-healthy things, except in testosterone improvement, but hopefully this book will change that antiquated thought! Keep in mind, however, if you lose weight on androgen deprivation therapy (ADT), it is one unique situation where weight loss does not cause an increase in testosterone, because the drug is intended to keep testosterone reduced, regardless of weight changes. But it will still improve your heart health! A win-win even in these unique situations!

Take Measure to Determine your Situation

How do you know if you're overweight or obese? People tend to underestimate their own weight, so a more objective measurement is needed. The standard used by medical practitioners is body mass index (BMI), which takes into account your weight and height. Another very good measure is waist circumference (WC). Often, it's a combination of these two that provides a more accurate picture of excess weight. (One of the best ways to find out exactly how much body fat you have is with a dual-energy x-ray absorptiometry, or DEXA scan—the same imaging test that tells someone if they have osteoporosis or not.)

Once you have your height and weight, it's easy to calculate your BMI. Use this formula: BMI = weight in pounds/height in inches 2 x 704 (or BMI = weight in kg/height in m^2, or you can just take your weight in kilograms and then divide it by your height in centimeters squared, and then multiply that entire result by 10,000.)

There are plenty of BMI calculators online, and they work much faster than doing your own calculation. Based on the number you get, you can categorize your weight as underweight, normal, overweight, or obese (see table). The catch with BMI is that it doesn't distinguish between lean mass—muscle, bones, organs, etc.—and fat. The more muscular you are (like athletes or me, in my mind), the higher your BMI will be, but that doesn't necessarily mean you're overweight. That's why using WC in addition to BMI is more accurate than using just one or the other. BMI is criticized all the time because it overlooks muscle mass but the average person walking around with a BMI of 30 or more (the obese category) often needs to lose some weight to improve their heart healthy numbers. On average, BMI performs well.

WC can be measured easily with a tape measure. Stand tall and find the top of your hip bones at the sides of your waist (not toward the front of the hips). Next poke around and find the bottom of your rib cage at the side. Exhale normally and place the tape measure around your waist midway between these points (it will be near the level of your belly button but probably not exactly at it). Take two normal breaths and on the exhale of the second breath tighten the tape measure so it's snug and straight and not digging into the skin. This will give you your waist circumference.

Why should you care about your waist size? Fat that accumulates around your middle near the skin is called "subcutaneous fat." There is also the more concerning type known as "visceral fat" especially deeper in the body, which can accumulate around and even inside your organs, such as the liver, pancreas, heart and even the leg, arm and other muscle tissues of the body making them less effective at working optimally for you. Excess fatty tissue can even settle within and around the prostate gland. In fact, researchers have preliminarily found that greater amounts of adipose tissue around the prostate ("periprostatic fat") could be associated with more unfavorable prostate cancer. This adipose tissue, could at least theoretically, secrete compounds that act almost like a fertilizer, ultimately helping unhealthy or malignant cells in the prostate grow and move to other parts of the body.

So, essentially excess adipose tissue reduces the efficacy of different body sites to work optimally and increases your risk of developing obesity-related conditions, such as diabetes, high blood pressure, coronary artery disease and non-alcoholic fatty liver disease (NAFLD, which will probably be the number one cause of liver transplant in the next generation). Again, we recognize the fact that it's very hard to lose weight or inches around the waist and keep it off long-term. And since some prostate cancer treatments make it even harder to lose excess fat there is no more important B to start with than Belly/BMI.

Body Mass Index (BMI) and Waist Circumference (WC) Values for Women and Men

BMI	Classification
Less than 18.5	Underweight
18.5 – 24.9	Normal weight
25 – 29.9	Overweight
30 or more	Obese

WC	Classification
Less than 35 in (89 cm) in men	Normal
35 to 39 in (89 to 99 cm) in men	Overweight
40 in or more (100 cm or more) in men	Obese
Less than 32.5 in (83 cm) in women	Normal
32.5 to 36 in (82.5–91.5 cm) in women	Overweight
37 in or more (94 cm or more) in women	Obese

Note: *Opinions may vary slightly for WC in terms of what is considered overweight or obese, but in general, these numbers are a good guide or starting point. Another measurement called the "waist-to-hip ratio" or WHR, can help clarify your weight picture. Lower WHR values tend to indicate better potential heart health (ask your healthcare team about it).*

If Your Clothes Could Talk

Perhaps the most simplistic measure of weight and whether you're gaining or losing is your clothing. Are your jeans getting tighter? If your pants/dresses/shirts are feeling less roomy, or primarily the waist size of your pants is increasing, unless you're adding lots of muscle, it's a sign that your weight or waist might need some attention.

PW Lifestyle Empowerment Moment

"If Your Prostate Could Talk"

The prostate in many men will increase in size if their weight or waist size increases a small or large amount, so one way to prevent your prostate from getting larger and causing urinary problems is to maintain a healthy weight/waist or even lose some weight/waist. Recent evidence suggests in some men their urinary symptoms get better and prostate size could decrease with some weight loss.

PW Lifestyle Empowerment Moment

First Step: Lifestyle Changes Change Lives

We've talked about how gaining weight or waist size can cause head-to-toe problems, but we also briefly discussed how losing weight and/or belly fat can reduce your risk of countless diseases and possibly improve your response to medical treatment. When it comes to numerous autoimmune conditions, some cancers and heart disease, clinical studies are demonstrating the potential for a greater chance of remission and response to treatment with healthy weight loss. Regardless, lifestyle changes can reduce the side effects of prostate cancer treatment!

It's also well accepted that lifestyle changes—eating better, exercising, improving sleep—can reduce weight/waist for many individuals, enough in some cases to improve the impact certain heart-healthy medications (such as those for cholesterol, high blood pressure, high blood sugar, etc.). Lifestyle changes can also help ensure that you only need the lowest dosage of a heart healthy medication in many situations, which is when the least amount of side effects occur. Even when medications or surgery is needed for weight loss, lifestyle changes increase the chances that the medications or surgery are effective long-term. In other words, lifestyle changes can change lives and moving this B in the right direction is the first step toward making gigantic leaps for your overall health.

Second Step: Medication for weight loss used to be a major problem.

Not anymore. Please ask your healthcare team!

Recent research suggests a variety of medications, especially those used for pre-diabetes or type 2 diabetes could result in substantial and potentially heart healthy weight loss for some individuals. For example, metformin has been used to help people lose small-to-moderate amounts of weight, but the newer prescription medications ("GLP-1 agonists"), such as "semaglutide," have resulted in significant, heart-healthy weight loss (thus far). In fact, the weight loss for many individuals using these medications have closely mirrored what has been observed for some weight loss surgeries (10-15% body weight loss) after two years. However, these medications are not without a few "catches," including cost, insurance coverage, and the need to continuously take it as a self-administered injection, or a pill in some cases. More testing in cancer patients is also immediately needed. Some gastrointestinal side effects may also occur, at least temporarily, in many people. Still, the options in this area are getting better and safer. While many past medications and even supplements helped people lose weight, they also caused heart rate and/or blood pressure to go up and they ended up being heart unhealthy, which is why many of them were permanently removed from the market.

Today, things appear to be very different. So, if you need some assistance with weight loss through a medical treatment then talk to your medical team ASAP about today's safer and more effective options. If you go on a medication, such as semaglutide or metformin, and some or most your 5Bs get better then you and your medical team can feel better knowing this medication is working for you. There is also the option of surgical weight loss, but this should be a discussion between you and your healthcare team, especially when all the other options have not worked long-term, and the weight you are carrying is life-threatening. You should also be fully educated on the pros and cons of these surgical procedures. In fact, any weight loss intervention, dietary or other lifestyle changes, fad diets, alternative treatments, commercial programs, weight loss clinics, etc. should be discussed with your healthcare team so you can learn about the latest and greatest, and no so great information.

PW Lifestyle Empowerment Moment

Extra bird seed you do not need.

Weight loss is so hard! Again, if anyone tells you it's not difficult then they probably live on another planet! Often, I will be on a lecture podium with a single 10-to-20-pound (approximately 5-10 kg) bag of bird seed, and then I will ask for any volunteers to come up and carry the bag with them the rest of the day. This is usually followed by strange looks from the audience. No volunteers?! Holding this bag for just five minutes is difficult (try it sometime—no kidding here). So just imagine how hard the human body struggles to handle and distribute this excess weight on the bones, organs, and other parts of the human body! This is exactly what happens when we gain excess weight or waist size— the body struggles to place it somewhere and when it does something else gets compromised in the process of storing this extra weight. The bag of bird seed is a visualization technique I use when someone thinks of lifestyle changes and the benefits of even a small amount of weight loss. The rare volunteer who decides to hold and then let go of an actual bird seed bag after only a few minutes of walking around with it feels not only lighter, but can also breathe easier, and just feels better.

The human body functions from head-to-toe more efficiently when someone removes "excess bird seed" (adipose tissue) from their liver, prostate, penis, pancreas, brain, etc. Again, we understand that it can be very hard to lose weight, but your body will reward you in countless ways if you are able to do this in the short- or long-term. Some of the ways it rewards you can be illustrated by the other 5 Bs and the bonus Bs! Better sleep, lower blood pressure, cholesterol, and blood sugar, more energy, better urinary function, better immune health (as we learned from the COVID-19 pandemic), improved sexual health, improved efficacy of some of the medications you're taking...I think you get the idea! Working with your healthcare team you can do this! Lose just a little bit of bird seed, and then watch the rest of your body fly in numerous positive directions you never dreamed of! Ok, that was a bit corny, but I had to end this chapter on a dramatic, powerful, and honest note!

Appendix 2—The Second B = Blood Cholesterol

Cholesterol Healthy = Head-to-Toe Healthier

High cholesterol levels have been associated with an increased risk of numerous medical conditions, including cardiovascular disease (CVD), certain eye diseases, dementia, prostate enlargement/urinary complications, more aggressive prostate cancer, recurrent prostate cancer, and sexual health issues (i.e., erectile dysfunction, female sexual dysfunction). It may also worsen countless other seemingly diverse health problems. For example, new research is looking into lowering high cholesterol levels, along with using standard of care medications, as another way to prevent migraine headaches. The culprit may be high levels of LDL (bad) cholesterol and/or triglycerides, which can increase inflammation in the body, and therefore contribute to migraines, as well as other conditions related to inflammation.

When discussing cholesterol, it's good to begin with a quick review. A standard fasting blood cholesterol test consists of the following:

- Total cholesterol (TC)
- Low-density lipoproteins (LDL or "bad" cholesterol)
- High-density lipoproteins (HDL or "good" cholesterol)
- Triglycerides or TG (fat in the blood)

PW Lifestyle Empowerment Moment

To fast or not to fast—that is the question. The answer: Fast for the cholesterol, glucose, and testosterone tests.

Although some argue you don't need to fast anymore to get accurate results on your cholesterol test the truth is triglycerides (fat in the blood) and/or glucose (sugar) levels can increase with a meal. Since many people today have high triglycerides and/or glucose, these numbers can jump to even higher levels without fasting. If this happens, you'll be asked to fast and retest anyway. Also, many healthcare providers monitoring men with prostate cancer, as well as other male patients, will occasionally look at a man's testosterone blood test to determine how he's doing. Recently, some notable medical groups are suggesting patients should fast before their testosterone blood test, because a meal can result in a significant temporary drop in your testosterone level. This could result in some men being diagnosed with low testosterone, when they do not carry such a low level (due to a temporary reduction caused by food). Also, if you're like most people, you get all your blood tests at one time or place (not just one isolated cholesterol test). If you're getting your cholesterol, glucose, testosterone, and multiple other blood tests at the same time, why not just end the uncertainty and extra potential lab visit and simply fast before your next blood test? Thank you. (Okay, time to get off my soapbox and return to our regularly scheduled book.)

Best cholesterol numbers for better heart health

For many years, healthcare professionals have encouraged patients to try to achieve "ideal" cholesterol numbers to prevent CVD and other health issues, as well as achieve better overall health. The following table shows where you stand for each aspect of cholesterol.

Cholesterol Numbers—What they mean and potential goals to work on with your healthcare team.	
LDL	**What It Means**
Less than 70 mg/dL (<1.81 mmol/L)	Ideal for people who have established CVD or are at high risk for a cardiac event.
Less than 100 mg/dL (< 2.59 mmol/L)	Optimal

100–129 mg/dL (2.59–3.34 mmol/L)	Nearly optimal
130–159 mg/dL (3.37–4.12 mmol/L)	Borderline high
160–189 mg/dL (4.14–4.90 mmol/L)	High
190 mg/dL or higher (4.92 mmol/L or higher)	Very high
HDL	**What It Means**
60 mg/dL or higher (1.55 mmol/L or higher)	Optimal
40–59 mg/dL (1.04–1.53 mmol/L)	Normal
Less than 40 mg/dL (< 1.04 mmol/L)	Too low
Triglycerides (TG)	**What It Means**
Less than 100 mg/dL (< 1.13 mmol/L)	Ideal (technically, this is "Moyad ideal")
Less than 150 mg/dL (< 1.69 mmol/L)	Normal
150–199 mg/dL (1.70-2.25 mmol/L)	Borderline high
200–499 mg/dL (2.26-5.64 mmol/L)	High
500 mg/dL or higher (5.65 mmol/L or higher)	Very high

Total Cholesterol (TC)	What It Means
Less than 160 mg/dL (< 4.14 mmol/L)	Optimal
160–200 mg/dL (4.14–5.16 mmol/L)	Desirable
201–238 mg/dL (5.17–6.19 mmol/L)	Borderline high
240 mg/dL or higher (6.20 mmol/L or higher)	High

Note: *To convert mg/dL of TC, HDL, or LDL to mmol/L, divide the number by 38.67; to go from mmol/L to mg/dL, multiply by 38.67. To convert mg/dL of TG to mmol/L, divide by 88.57; to go from mmol/L to mg/dL, multiply by 88.57. General weight gain, including from ADT or other medications could increase triglycerides (another barometer of metabolic health by itself), especially as adipose tissue increases. Excessive amounts of calories from carbohydrates ("bad carbs" or "sugars") could also increase triglycerides, drop HDL, and increase the risk of numerous other conditions such as fatty liver disease.*

Bonus: Apo B Blood Test(s) can also assist in predicting cardiovascular risk.

There is another blood test that is gaining popularity because it collectively measures most of the well-known and lesser-known cholesterol or lipoprotein numbers (e.g., LDL, IDL, VLDL, lipoprotein a-form or type of LDL, non-HDL cholesterol) you want to have on the lower end to reduce your risk of CVD. This blood test is called "Apo B," and you should talk to your healthcare team about it because increasing evidence suggests it may be one of the best blood tests available to predict risk along with the other traditional numbers mentioned in the table (LDL, TG, TC, etc.). Often the LDL is a good enough predictor of the level of bad guys in your blood, but the Apo B test may provide a more complete picture. Additionally, a test called "Apo A" collectively measures most of the numbers you want to have on the higher end (HDL or types of HDL), and you can also talk to your healthcare team about this test. These tests can help in some (not all) situations to see if there is more you and your healthcare team can do to reduce your risk of CVD.

The cholesterol conundrum ("catch"), but you can still collect more puzzle pieces.

Some studies suggest up to 50 percent of the first-time heart attacks occur in people who have "normal" cholesterol levels, so it's obvious that cholesterol alone isn't an accurate enough risk assessment tool—but it's still important. Recently, experts have developed new assessments that provide enhanced information about heart disease and stroke risk, which go beyond the traditional cholesterol numbers. For example, CT-based coronary calcium scoring ("CAC"), or in some special cases a CT-based coronary angiogram (CTA), which are non-invasive picture tests, are often used to assess risk more accurately. However, you should talk to your healthcare team to see if you qualify for these or other special tests (e.g., an EKG app on your phone) for cardiovascular disease (CVD) detection. (This is also mentioned in the Bonus B section for emphasis.)

To get a clearer, faster and simpler idea at home of where you stand that goes beyond just your cholesterol, you can go to cvriskcalculator.com and fill out a quick, easy risk assessment that you can discuss with your healthcare team on your next visit. This and two other commonly used risk calculators, the Framingham Coronary Heart Disease Risk Score, and the Systematic Coronary Risk Evaluation (SCORE), are used in clinics around the world. (Ask your physician which one they prefer to use.) The cvriskcalculator.com, from the American College of Cardiology/ American Heart Association, calculates an estimated risk (higher is more concerning) over time—usually 10 years—and suggests some medications you may qualify for right now based on that risk, such as cholesterol-lowering medications. They also have many wonderful lifestyle recommendations on these sites that you can institute to boost heart health.

The good news is if you do qualify for conventional cholesterol-lowering medicines, such as statins, they are also anti-inflammatory, primarily generic and cost effective. They can be very helpful for people who aren't able to reduce their CVD risk enough with realistic, moderate and practical lifestyle changes. Which leads me to...

PW Lifestyle Empowerment Moment

Reducing your LDL and triglycerides and improving your HDL is possible for many individuals today with a combination of moderate dietary changes, exercise, weight loss, and possibly (but not necessarily) medical treatment. Regular exercise is still one of the best ways to increase HDL and losing just a small amount of weight or changing your diet can significantly lower triglycerides and LDL (plus lower your blood pressure and blood sugar), while also raising HDL. In fact, blood cholesterol was one of the first risk measurements where experts realized lifestyle changes could be so powerful. Some people can avoid medication altogether, or at least reduce their dosages or improve the effectiveness of their medications, with lifestyle changes alone.

PW Lifestyle Empowerment Moment

First Step: Lifestyle Changes Change Lives—You are your own TV infomercial testimonial.

If you're wondering whether your heart-healthy lifestyle choices are paying off, give yourself just two to three months with your new habits and then see how your retested numbers compare to your old ones. The beauty of this second B, as in the other B's, is that it responds quickly to lifestyle changes and/or can improve the efficacy of your cholesterol lowering medication, as well as potentially other medications. When people see the dramatic changes in their B numbers after just three to six months with lifestyle changes, they become their own infomercial testimonial—which means they can tell others what they did, which not only helps other people, but is also self-motivational because of the tangible results. In other words, be your own "before" and "after" commercial. Now you know why TV health testimonials are so powerful (whether you agree with them or not), because they inspire others to make changes. People love the "before" and "after" pictures, but we also love the before and after B numbers (as we should)!

Second Step: Not able to tolerate a statin medication? Nocebo? No problem.

In the past, some people were not able to tolerate their statin or cholesterol lowering drug because it caused muscle and/or joint issues or other problems. However, more extensive research from clinical trials demonstrated that only a small percentage of these issues were due to the drug itself. It turns out daily aches and pains from a variety of causes, along with an avalanche of negative perceptions and commentary on the internet about these drugs, before even taking them, encouraged or promoted the feeling that something was wrong when taking them. This is known as the "nocebo" (aka "I will harm") effect, which is opposite of the placebo (aka "I will please") effect. Nocebo causes some people to believe they are experiencing a problem or side effect, because they have been inundated with what could go wrong. Therefore, it's not difficult to imagine that something negative is occurring even when nothing is wrong. In some cases, positive thinking can be powerful medicine to alleviate discomfort, but so is negative thinking, which can encourage discomfort.

However, there are still some people who experience real side effects from these drugs. Statins are some of the most common drugs on the planet, which means there are bound to be some people who are sensitive to them. The good news is there are so many generic statin options today, that dosages, frequency, and even the type of statin drug can be switched several or many times (working with your healthcare team) until you find one that fits you, sans side effects of course. Still, what if you are the rare case where none of these drugs can be tolerated? No worries, lets' review the incredible number of options you have today (including statins). Please keep in mind if you can lower your cholesterol, even a little with lifestyle, it still translates into needing a lower dose of a cholesterol lowering medication, so lifestyle changes are as important as ever when taking any of these drugs.

So many amazing pills and injectable ways to solve your cholesterol puzzle today—along with lifestyle changes of course!

Statins (numerous cheap options now available)
Statins continue to drop in price (due to so many generics) and continue to have the most research to suggest they can reduce the risk of CVD. Statins can lower LDL cholesterol levels between 20 and 60 percent, depending on the patient. They are also being studied now to determine if they lower the risk of prostate cancer recurrence after treatment, or even delay or prevent the transition from hormone sensitive prostate cancer to CRPC (castrate

resistant prostate cancer). Since there are so many generic options today, if one doesn't work well, you can talk to your healthcare team about trying a different one. Keep in mind that fluvastatin (Lescol), pitavastatin (Livalo), pravastatin (Pravachol), and rosuvastatin (Crestor) can be combined with grapefruit/grapefruit juice without a negative drug interaction. However, lovastatin (Mevocor), simvastatin (Zocor, Vytorin), and atorvastatin (Lipitor) can interact negatively with grapefruit and increase the risk of side effects. This is usually more problematic at the higher dosages of these medications.

Bempedoic acid (new pill)
This is a newer pill (drug) approved in some countries, such as the U.S. and the European Union.

Somewhat like statins, "Bempedoic acid" (Nexletol) also blocks part of the cholesterol producing pathway but is known as a "citrate lyase inhibitor" and can lower LDL cholesterol by about 20%. It may be a good option for people who truly cannot tolerate statin medications. In some cases, it can be combined with ezetimibe.

Ezetimibe (older pill)
"Ezetimibe" can be taken along with a statin or bempedoic acid in some cases. This pill (drug) reduces the intestinal absorption of cholesterol and can further reduce LDL cholesterol by 10-20%. In rare cases, ezetimibe can also be taken by itself to reduce LDL, but the data to support this is not as strong.

Omega-3/Fish Oil (prescription does have FDA approval, but...?)
Other pill options such as omega-3 or "fish oil" prescription drugs can help to lower high triglycerides and can also be taken along with a statin drug, but the data to support their use alone for cholesterol reduction is not strong. In addition, taking higher dosages of fish oil could raise LDL cholesterol in some cases, and cause other issues (e.g., blood thinning). Fish oil is not approved to lower LDL cholesterol (only triglycerides).

PCSK9 inhibitors—New "game changing" kids on the block!

"PCSK9 inhibitors" (aka "proprotein convertase subtilisin/kexin type 9 inhibitors") are injectable (usually once every two or four weeks) human monoclonal antibody medications you can give yourself at home. They are one of the most exciting potential advances in the field of CVD reduction! PCSK-9 is a protein that helps to target the LDL receptor for degradation or removal. By inhibiting PCSK-9, a dramatic reduction in LDL can occur—in many cases up to 50-60%! The rate of side effects tends to be low with injection site redness (erythema) occurring in about 5% of patients and sometimes malaise or feeling not well for a day or two after the injection. These drugs can also be combined with statins in some cases. Currently, the real issue with these medications is the high cost and lack of coverage by insurance, but both are getting a little better. Additionally, a PCSK9 inhibitor pill is being researched now and may be available in the future. While a pill form may lower costs, many patients like the option of an injection because it takes seconds to administer and then you're done for at least two weeks. Alirocumab (Praluent) and evolocumab (Repatha) are two of the more commonly known drugs in this class.

Another injection known as "inclisiran" (Leqvio) works by a slightly different mechanism (small interfering RNA or siRNA to also impact PCSK9) and has been shown to reduce LDL by 50% in some patients versus a placebo. Only two to three injections are needed per year (initial dose, second dose three months later and then every six months after that)! This class of drugs is currently only an option for a select group of patients, but it's one to watch because it's gaining a lot of attention.

Note: *There are other older medications that can lower cholesterol (bile acid sequestrants, fibrates, etc.), but this should be a discussion between you and your healthcare team.*

Quick Table Review to Show Your Healthcare Team

Please keep in mind the greater the dedication to lifestyle changes then the lower the dosage of the drug needed for many people, which means an even lesser rate of the already low risk of side effects from these medications!

Medication/Drug Class (so many options today)	LDL ("bad cholesterol") Reduction	Major Potential Side Effects
Statins (first-line therapy) • Atorvastatin • Lovastatin • Pitavastatin • Pravastatin • Simvastatin • Rosuvastatin *(Note: all options are in the form of pills. Grapefruit can possibly interact with atorvastatin, lovastatin or simvastatin.)*	40-60% at the higher intensity dosages, but with lifestyle changes lower dosages are often needed to achieve your goal!	• Myalgias—muscle issues (5-10%) • Rhabdomyolysis—serious medical condition from muscle breakdown (less than 1 out of 10,000) • Liver Function Test (LFT) increases (1%-2%) • New diagnosis of diabetes mellitus (1 to 3 out of every 10,000 annually)
Bempedoic Acid (pill)	20% at recommended dosages, and do not forget your lifestyle changes!	• Myalgia (1%-2% and less than placebo in some clinical studies)
Ezetimibe	20% at 10 mg daily dose, and do not forget your lifestyle changes!	• Myalgias (2-3%) • LFT increase (1%) • Diarrhea, abdominal discomfort

PCSK9 Inhibitors • Alirocumab (Praluent) • Evolocumab (Repatha) (a subcutaneous injection-every 2 weeks or monthly—can be done at home)	50-60% at recommended dosages in untreated and statin-treated patients, and do not forget your lifestyle changes!	• Injection site erythema/redness (5%-10%), • Malaise (1%-2%)

Notes:

- Inclisiran (Leqvio) is another newer type of PCSK9 inhibitor, which should also be a more widely available injectable option in the future and do not forget your lifestyle changes!

- Fish oil does not lower LDL cholesterol significantly enough to compete with the medications in the table, but some prescription forms such as icosapent ethyl (EPA only product) can reduce triglycerides by 20-40%. However, it could also increase the risk of new-onset atrial fibrillation at higher dosages in a small percentage of people (1%-2%). Also, some forms of fish oil (with EPA & DHA) could paradoxically increase LDL levels at higher dosages. (The potential for lower dosages of fish oil pills to prevent other non-cardiovascular conditions can be found in the supplement chapter.).

- Supplements to reduce cholesterol are no longer as exciting because the prescription medication category has become so diverse, more reliable, smaller pill sizes/dosage, and are often lower in cost (especially statins). Also, the need for coenzyme Q10 supplements to reduce the risk of side effects from statins is also questionable and taking another pill for a rare side effect is not only costly, but unnecessary for many people because they can be switched to something today that causes minimal-to-no side effects.

Cholesterol lowering in prostate cancer is very hot right now!

There are countless clinical trials ongoing to determine what role, if any, statins, and other cholesterol lowering medications (especially PCSK9 inhibitors) have within prostate cancer. Recently, research has suggested they could lower the risk of being diagnosed with non-aggressive prostate cancer (overdiagnosis). They are also being studied to reduce the risk of cancer returning after conventional treatment or slowing the progression of prostate cancer with conventional treatment. It is now known for example, they appear to reduce the production of some adrenal androgens, and/or discourage them from reaching cancer cells so they cannot fuel these cells. For example, researchers are trying to determine if it could further improve the response to ADT (androgen deprivation treatment) as some preliminary studies have suggested, or reduce some of the side effects from it, and other treatments.

Still, what if all this research fails to show a real benefit regarding prostate cancer? The fact that these medications increase the probability of living longer in some men with prostate cancer by reducing their risk of cardiovascular disease/events, which is the number one cause of death in prostate cancer patients, is reason enough to have a discussion with your healthcare team about achieving the second B—healthy blood cholesterol!

Additionally, lifestyle changes and cholesterol lowering medications could reduce the risk of cardiovascular issues in men on ADT and those taking anti-androgen prostate cancer drugs, which are associated with an additional increased risk of cardiovascular problems in some patients—so they have a role to play in prostate cancer regardless of how one looks at it. Statins (and other cholesterol lowering medications) also reduce inflammation, help unstable plaques in the arteries become more stable so they cannot trigger a cardiovascular event, such as a heart attack or stroke, and have some blood thinning properties. And, being monitored by your healthcare team while you're taking statins can reduce the risk of side effects from them. So, please "Be" excited about lowering this B!

Appendix 3—The Third B = Blood Pressure

The Most Important Inaccurate Measurement?

Here is something that might really surprise you—blood pressure (BP) is the most important and simplest heart-healthy measurement, but it's also the most inaccurately measured heart-healthy barometer of all those discussed in this promoting wellness book! Why? Because so many factors can falsely increase or decrease the number. High blood pressure (hypertension) is a scary epidemic with more than half the population currently living with this condition. This epidemic is partially due to weight gain and other lifestyle factors (e.g., stress, inactivity, increased alcohol intake), combined with the inflammation that occurs with heart-unhealthy changes. Regardless of the cause, now is the time to accurately measure your BP and monitor it regularly to determine if your diet and/or other lifestyle changes, along with medication, if needed, is working.

> ### PW Lifestyle Empowerment Moment
>
> What is arguably the most important thing you can do before you get a blood pressure (BP) reading? Empty your bladder! Yes, empty your bladder even if you think you do not need to use the bathroom! Having a full bladder can temporarily, but dramatically increase your blood pressure. (More on this later.)

High blood pressure loves to quietly damage everything in its path.

Most heart attacks, strokes, and even initial heart failure occur in individuals with high blood pressure (hypertension). In fact, high blood pressure is becoming the most common risk factor for cardiovascular disease (CVD). Some more recent studies are now showing that up to 60-70% of the general adult population has an abnormally high blood pressure. So, what specifically is an abnormally high blood pressure? Well, times have changed and so have the blood pressure guidelines based on the latest research—and this is a very good thing since we need more awareness, and high blood pressure is so destructive to the entire body from the head-to-toes.

Uncontrolled long-term hypertension injures or damages everything in its path, including ears (hearing), eyes, memory (brain tissue), sexual function, arteries/blood vessels high and low (peripheral artery disease), heart (arrhythmias, failure), kidneys, bone health (new research), circulation, and more. I think you get the idea of why it's so problematic! What's more, high blood pressure is often silent or subtle during its initial destruction of different body parts, which is why more awareness is always needed. Many prostate cancer treatments, or medications such as ADT or anti-androgen drugs are associated with BP increases in some patients, which is another of the many reasons this chapter is so very necessary! For example, abiraterone pills (often combined with ADT) can cause an increase in BP soon after starting treatment, which is why healthcare teams usually prescribe another pill with it to reduce the risk of BP increasing side effects!

Blood Pressure (BP) Categories

Blood Pressure (BP) Diagnosis/Category	Systolic (mm Hg) BP (upper #)	AND/OR	Diastolic (mm Hg) BP (lower #)
Normal	Less than 120	AND	Less than 80
Elevated	120-129	AND	Less than 80
High Blood Pressure-Hypertension-Stage 1	130-139	OR	80-89

High Blood Pressure-Hypertension-Stage 2	140 or Higher	OR	90 or Higher
Hypertensive Crisis (consult your doctor immediately)	Higher Than 180	AND/OR	Higher Than 120

Source: *American Heart Association/American Stroke Association (they are awesome!)*

Your complete guide to accurately measuring your own BP.

Blood pressure (BP) is a critical measurement and getting an accurate measurement especially when done once a year in an office or at home is not easy. The problem is that so many things can impact your BP, causing the number to look artificially high and even artificially low. The one factor that always seems to get the most attention is referred to as "white-coat hypertension" or the fear of going to the physician's office, which can cause a temporary increase in blood pressure due to stress. Of course, there are many other factors that can temporarily impact blood pressure, including those listed in the following table.

As mentioned in the PW Empowerment Moment, one of the best things you can do to get an accurate blood pressure reading is to simply empty your bladder before your blood pressure is measured (even if you think you do not need to use the bathroom, please try to empty it). A bladder that is partially full or full can cause a temporary large jump in your numbers due to the back pressure it can put on the kidneys, which then temporarily increases the pressure in other areas of the body. This pressure releases a variety of compounds which cause arteries to constrict and BP to register as higher than normal. The impact of urine in the bladder affects some people more than others during the BP measurement. Interestingly, one class of blood pressure medications—diuretics—work by allowing you to get rid of excess fluid in the body to help reduce BP. In other words, reducing excess amounts of fluid in the body reduces blood pressure, and what is one thing that can dramatically increase the amount of fluid in the body? Sodium in excess! (More on this later.)

Factors That Can Cause Temporary Blood Pressure Changes

(Wow, there are a lot of things here, but like anything else, when you review this list several times it will become second nature to do these things whenever you take your BP, or when someone takes it for you.*)

Patient Behavior or Situation	Potential Blood Pressure Increase
A full or distended bladder	10-15 mm Hg
Engaged in a conversation during the BP reading, or not having at least 5 minutes of quiet time before the measurement	10-15 mm Hg
BP cuff over clothing, cuff size issues, or pulling up sleeve instead of removing your shirt/sleeve (you want a "naked/bare" arm when measuring) or leaving on one sleeve layer not pulled-up. (Pulled-up sleeve creates a tourniquet effect that can act like a tight cuff and falsely increase BP.)	10-40 mm Hg Cuff around arm is too small before inflated (tight) = higher BP. Cuff too big (loose) = lower BP. Cuff should ideally be placed over bare skin because sleeves can make it hard to position the cuff in some cases and cause false increases.
Unsupported back and/or feet and/or arm	5-10 mm Hg
Crossed legs	2-8 mm Hg

Arm with blood pressure cuff is not supported and not at the level of your heart when measurement is taken, or cuff is too small. Here are the recommended cuff sizes after measuring your mid-upper arm circumference (cm or inches=in).** Small Adult = 22-26 cm (8.7-10.2 inches) Adult = 27-34 cm (10.6-13.4 inches) Large Adult = 35-44 cm (13.8-17.3 inches) Extra Large Adult = 45-52 cm (17.7-20.5 inches)	Variable increases (approximately **10 mm Hg**) and even decreases. (If upper arm is below the level of the heart, it can cause false increases in BP reading. If arm is above heart level, then the reading can be falsely low. Either situation increases or decreases BP 2 mm Hg for every inch above or below the heart level.). Cuff sizes are either printed on the cuff itself, device manual, or BP container/box.
Ingestion of caffeine, nicotine from any tobacco products within the past 30-60 minutes.	Variable increases & decreases in some select cases***
Exertion, brisk walking, running, lifting, or other exercise 30-60 minutes before the measurement.	Variable increases & decreases in some select cases***
Stress/anxiety right before the measurement, and talking during measurement or within several minutes before the measurement.	Variable increases

*Source: *AMA News and AHA Scientific Statement*

**Note: *Mid-upper arm can be found by measuring the length of the arm between the first part of the bony protuberances on shoulder (called "acromion process"), and the bony protuberance at elbow (called the "olecranon process"), and then divide the distance in half to find the exact location of your mid-upper arm. Next, you can wrap the tape measure around the mid-upper arm, and this will give you the arm circumference measurement, which then can tell you if you need a small adult, adult, large adult, or extra-large adult cuff size on your BP device.*

***Note:** When someone is dependent or addicted to a specific drug substance, such as nicotine and/or alcohol then abrupt withdrawal from that substance could cause large temporary increases in BP (talk to your medical team about safely quitting any drug addiction). However, safely quitting these substances could eventually result in a wonderful and beneficial long-term reduction in BP. Also, exercise can cause BP increases during and right after the exercise, whereas for some time after exercise then BP could drop and help with BP reductions long-term.*

Home is also where the accuracy is.

What is the most important way to get a consistently accurate blood pressure reading?

Buy your own validated for accuracy device and take your BP at home. As discussed, many people have elevated blood pressure readings when at a physician's office or other clinical setting due to stress. This issue can be solved by taking readings at home.

Talk to your healthcare team, which may include your pharmacist, about which blood pressure devices are the most tested, accurate, and clinically validated to use at home. Research continues to suggest blood pressure monitoring at home, when done properly, is as accurate or even more accurate in some cases than the blood pressures numbers obtained at your local healthcare center, but of course both are needed to ensure accuracy.

ABPM is the answer when there is no clear answer.

What if in the rare case my physician and I are not able to reach a consensus on what my most accurate average blood pressure is? If you and your physician are not able to somehow reach an accurate level or knowledge of what your blood pressure is (a rare, but important situation), then ask for a continuous 24-hour Ambulatory Blood Pressure Monitor (also known as "ABPM") to end the drama. ABPM is the gold standard of accuracy in those rare cases where home and clinic blood pressure readings are not consistent! You will have to wear this device for approximately one full day, during which it takes blood pressure readings continuously, even when you're sleeping.

Bonus BP Measuring Tips

Miscellaneous blood pressure tips to ensure accuracy:

- Try to take blood pressure readings at a similar time of day and then wait at least one minute after your first reading, and then take your BP again, and then again at least one minute later after the second reading because an average of three consecutive readings is helpful for overall accuracy. BP also usually fluctuates during the day, but morning and afternoon readings on the same day are helpful.

- Multiple readings over several months give the best accuracy.

- Initial or first-time reading with a home device or in an office should measure BP in both arms to make sure there is not a large variation that might suggest a cardiovascular problem. After that, occasionally still take readings in both arms. Additionally, recent evidence suggests measuring an occasional BP when lying down and then standing up should be reported to your healthcare team. Normally, BP can slightly drop upon standing, especially when moving from a lying down position to standing, so if your systolic number increases 6-7 mm Hg or more when standing recent research (HARVEST study) suggests a potential increased risk of a future cardiovascular event. This appears to be due to an increase in stress hormones upon standing (sympathetic overactivity), but more research is needed.

- Significantly warm or cold room temperature, background noise, or muscle tension can cause an artificial reading.

- Alcohol intake before the BP reading can also cause changes in BP

Fast review on how to get the most accurate BP for YOU

To summarize, next time you get a BP measurement, empty your bladder, avoid exercise, tobacco, and caffeine at least 30 minutes minimally to an hour before the reading. Relax with no talking or active listening for five minutes before the measurement and do not talk during the measurement. Sit up straight with your back supported, both feet flat on the ground and arm supported at or around heart level. Make sure the cuff is the right size and placed on your bare skin with sleeve/shirt removed (not rolled up), and again please remain quiet during the test. Also, keep in mind that at-home finger blood pressure and many wrist monitors have not been consistently accurate. Ideally, you want a blood pressure cuff to go around your upper arm for the most accurate measurement, but if an arm is too large for any accessible BP cuff, then a wrist device to measure BP could be obtained until the cuff issue is solved. Also, take an occasional BP measurement in both arms, and a BP from a lying to standing position, and then share all these recent measurements with your healthcare team at each visit. Wow! Now you can see why blood pressure measurements have the potential to be inaccurate, but this chapter should help change that (along with the American Medical Association or AMA and many other medical organizations that have dramatically raised awareness of this issue by investing in more education of healthcare professionals and the public).

"One and cannot be done"—again please also bring it home to home in on your true BP numbers!

BP is one of the most important health numbers, and yet many of us rely on ONE office visit, where ONE blood pressure reading is taken, to determine our health ONCE a year! If blood pressure is a concern due to your numbers or family history, again please consider buying your own validated for accuracy blood pressure monitoring device at a local pharmacy and take your own blood pressure several times a year (or even several times a month). Share your numbers with your healthcare team at your next visit and this will increase the chances that your readings are accurate. Interestingly, one of the most common ways doctors are now identifying those at risk for type 2 diabetes (apart from weight gain, family history, and diet) is by a consistent elevation in blood pressure, which can be an indication to order a blood sugar test.

PW Lifestyle Empowerment Moment

First Step: Lifestyle Changes Change Lives

DASH Diet was and still is a game changer along with other lifestyle advice!

Thanks to the DASH (Dietary Approaches to Stop Hypertension) diet*, clinical trials, and countless other studies, research has clearly demonstrated that for many people moderate lifestyle changes (change in diet and/or weight loss) work as well as many lower dosage blood pressure-lowering medications to reduce BP. Additionally, lifestyle changes can make many BP medications work better at lower dosages (where fewer side effects occur). What is also really empowering is just a two-point drop in individuals with high blood pressure can reduce the risk of death from stroke, heart disease, and all causes. Just two points! Lifestyle changes rule!

Interestingly, dietary potassium was one of the primary reasons the DASH diet was successful in lowering blood pressure—more than any other diet tested in large and well-done clinical trials. Still, if you increase your intake of dietary potassium from healthy whole unprocessed foods then other healthy compounds such as calcium, magnesium, and fiber come along for the ride, and many unhealthy compounds, such as sodium, and sugar, along with other bad carbs, fats and proteins are minimal or non-existent in those foods.

(*For more on the DASH diet, talk to a dietician recommended by your healthcare care team. More information is also provided throughout this book.)

Each (let us repeat that)—each individual lifestyle tip below could reduce blood pressure, but the more you can do the merrier for your BP!

Alcohol reduced or eliminated

(One of the most under-appreciated causes of high blood pressure—even occasional, moderate, and binge drinking can cause increases in BP)

Caloric quantity reduction

(Just 250-500 calories per day)

DASH diet. Please visit nhlbi.nih.gov/DASH

(Caloric quality improvements focusing on veggies, fruits, whole grains, beans, peas, nuts and seeds, along with fat-free or low-fat dairy, fish, and poultry. Limited use of vegetable oils. Avoids or reduces fatty meats, full-fat dairy, sodium, sugar sweetened beverages, and sweets. The diet is low in saturated and trans fats, with higher intakes of potassium, calcium, magnesium, fiber, and protein from healthy foods, while greatly reducing sodium intake.)

Exercise

(Especially aerobic, but also flexibility, and potentially strength training)

Medication reductions/changes (talk to your healthcare team)

(Pain relievers—NSAIDs such as ibuprofen/naproxen, and even other pills such as acetaminophen in large enough dosages can increase BP in some individuals, according to recent research. Also, many over the counter (OTC) decongestants such as ephedrine, pseudoephedrine, phenylephrine, naphazoline, and oxymetazoline can increase BP and heart rate. These compounds can also be found in some allergy pills—check labels carefully, especially ones that end in "-D" such as "Allegra-D, Claritin-D, Zyrtec-D." etc.)

(Also, fizzy or effervescent tablets and products can contain 100s of milligrams of sodium per single tablet and should be reduced, eliminated and substituted for a lower-to-no sodium option if possible.)

Potassium from plant-based heart healthy dietary sources increased

(Vegetables, fruits, beans, lentils, nuts, seeds, whole grains, etc.)

Sleep quality and quantity improved

(Six hours or less is BP unhealthy, while 7-8 hours is a good goal. Recent research also suggests the potential for improved weight loss with adequate sleep. Following other lifestyle advice in this table can also improve the quality of your sleep such as alcohol reduction/elimination, exercise, etc.)

Sodium (salt) reduction to 2,300 mg/day or in some cases 1,500 mg/day for those who are salt-sensitive

(Reduce or eliminate processed foods/snacks, such as chips, crackers, pretzels, popcorn, and snack mixes. In addition, breads & rolls, burritos & tacos, cheese, chicken, cold cuts & cured meats, restaurant food, pizza, eggs & omelets, sandwiches, soups,...can all be loaded with sodium. Be sure to check labels because there are major differences among similar products! Notice how the saltshaker was not mentioned because it usually contributes a small amount to the total, but if it's used often than switching to potassium chloride or salt substitute now has research it can be heart healthy and reduce the risk of stroke and other cardiovascular events—see the QQ dietary chapter.)

Stress reduction

(Stress releases hormones that increase blood pressure, and in fact the beta-blocker category of blood pressure drugs works by reducing the impact of your stress hormones! White coat hypertension is enough ample evidence by itself to show how stress can dramatically increase BP! Meditation and some breathing exercise devices such as RESPeRATE now have clinical evidence they can also help with BP reduction!)

Tobacco eliminated

Weight/Waist Loss

(Approximately a one-point BP drop for every two pounds lost! It's not unusual today for patients to lose a good deal of weight then reduce the dosage of their BP medications with their healthcare team. Lifestyle changes change lives!)

Note: *Many diets (not just DASH, although it has the most evidence) or lifestyle changes can reduce BP, but the list in the table above covers the major BP reducing methods to consider when following any program. Another tip, less often recommended, is being sensitive to substance abuse of any kind (talk to your healthcare team about it). Dependence or addiction causes many underappreciated issues including BP swings from high and low on a regular basis, which is heart unhealthy.*

Second Step: Many low-cost medications. Low-dosages of more than one type may work better and be safer than higher dosages of just one type of blood pressure reducing pill.

Interestingly, recent research suggests lifestyle changes combined with anti-hypertensive medications are more effective in preventing cardiovascular problems and reducing the risk of an early death (a true PW lifestyle empowerment moment) compared to just taking medication alone. Research also continues to suggest one of the best ways to control high blood pressure with medications is by using two or more different types/classes of drugs at lower dosages compared to just one type at a higher dosage. For example, there are now multiple classes of anti-hypertensive medications (e.g., ARBs, beta-blockers, calcium channel blockers, diuretics), each with their own pros and cons, but most are generic and can be potentially combined. Therefore, taking an effective medication should be a discussion between you and your healthcare team because it's easier today than ever before, and should also be more affordable.

There is another class of blood pressure drugs called "ACE inhibitors," but recent research continues to suggest the ARB class of medications are just as effective, but with less side effects. Regardless, the real point is that blood pressure drugs, along with lifestyle changes are lifesaving, easier than ever to take, and have a variety of low-cost options. These options should be discussed with your healthcare team, in terms of which one or ones are the best to try.

Blood pressure healthy = Urinary Health = Urinary Fitness

One of the most common classes of drugs being prescribed in the world today to help men urinate when they have prostate problems are called "alpha-blockers." These drugs were originally used to lower blood pressure and then research demonstrated a side benefit—men were able to urinate more effectively (less frequently) when they were taking them. Thus, many of the alpha-blockers prescribed today to help men with prostate or urination issues were derived from older blood pressure drugs! Heart healthy = urination healthy?! But wait there is more! Viagra and other drugs like it (known as "PDE-5 inhibitors") have been approved for erectile dysfunction (ED), but now some drugs in this class are also being used to improve urinary health in men with benign prostatic hyperplasia (BPH). Some of these drugs are also able to reduce or improve blood pressure in different parts of the body (such as the lungs). In other words, it's interesting how some medications in men's health, which can favorably impact blood pressure also have an ability to improve urinary fitness.

In fact, it's not just about medication. Research continues to demonstrate heart healthy lifestyle changes, including those that lower blood pressure (especially exercise) help men get up less at night to urinate (called "nocturia") and help empty the bladder more effectively. Yeah!

Appendix 4—The Fourth B = Blood Sugar

Blood Sugar Healthy = Head-to-Toe Healthier

Before we delve into this chapter, here are some tough, but true statistics for you to consider:

- Approximately one out of every 10 adults aged 20 years and older (10% of the population) have type 2 diabetes (diabetes mellitus).

- Diabetes is a major risk factor for cardiovascular disease (CVD) and stroke.

- Diabetes also increases the risk for numerous cancers and cancer recurrence after treatment.

- In young adults with type 2 diabetes, 10% are overweight and 80% are obese.

- Type 2 diabetes now accounts for 90-95% of all cases of diagnosed diabetes.

- Type 2 diabetes is the most common reason for nerve damage (neuropathy).

- Type 2 diabetes is one of the most common causes of kidney failure and blindness and is the most common cause of amputation.

- Blood sugar (glucose) control issues increased & still increases the risk of COVID-19 progression and severity.

- There are no obvious signs of prediabetes, which is characterized by an abnormally high blood sugar level, but not quite diabetes yet.

- Waist/weight gain before, during, and after prostate cancer treatment can be associated with an increase in the risk of pre-diabetes, type 2 diabetes, or making these existing situations worse.

Hemoglobin A1c is getting more attention for a reason.

Blood sugar is commonly measured to determine if someone has normal blood sugar, prediabetes, or diabetes. There are several tests normally used to monitor blood sugar levels, including fasting and random blood sugar test. However, the Hemoglobin A1c (HgbA1c) test provides a three-month average of blood sugar levels. This test might be appropriate if preliminary screenings are of concern. Overall, the HghA1c is probably the most accurate test to determine if you have normal blood sugar, are prediabetic, or have type-2 diabetes. This test is based on the attachment of glucose (sugar) to hemoglobin, the protein in red blood cells that carries oxygen. Because the lifespan of a red blood cell is roughly three months, this test tells you and your healthcare team what percentage of your hemoglobin A is "coated with sugar" (glycated). If you are concerned about your blood sugar, ask your healthcare team for more information about this test.

The following table will give you a good overview of what numbers suggest normal, prediabetes, and type 2 diabetes.

Blood Sugar Test	Normal Level	Prediabetes	Type 2 Diabetes
Fasting blood sugar	99 mg/dl (5.5 mmol/L) or lower	100-125 mg/dl (5.6-6.9 mmol/L)	126 mg/dl (7.0 mmol/L) or higher
Hemoglobin A1c (average blood sugar over past 2-3 months)	5.6% or lower	5.7% to 6.4%	6.5% or greater
Random blood sugar test	139 mg/dl (7.7 mmol/L) or lower	140-199 mg/dl (7.8-11.0 mmol/L)	200 mg/dl (11.1 mmol/L) or higher with common diabetes symptoms
Oral glucose tolerance test (OGTT)	140 mg/dl (7.7 mmol/L) or lower	140-199 mg/dl (7.8-11.0 mmol/L)	200 mg/dl (11.1 mmol/L) or higher

Note: *Many of these tests should be repeated if abnormal to ensure an accurate result.*

Also, high dosages (in the range of 1000 mg or more) of some supplements taken during the time of the hemoglobin A1c test could falsely increase or decrease the result. Higher supplemental dosages of vitamin E (false decrease) and vitamin C (false increase or decrease based on specific type of HgbA1c lab test utilized) are the ones associated with the greater preliminary concern. Low blood levels of B12, folate, or iron can result in an anemia that could also cause a false increase in HgBA1c. Higher doses of supplemental vitamin C could also falsely alter the results of other glucose tests from preliminary studies. Talk to your healthcare team about the latest information on what can and cannot impact your blood tests. Most medical professionals will not encourage mega-doses of these supplements, in any case, because vitamin E in high dosages was associated with a higher risk of prostate cancer in the famous SELECT trial, and mega-dosages of vitamin C could increase the risk of kidney stones in some patients.

PW Lifestyle Empowerment Moment

"Sugar feeds cancer?" Not exactly—Please focus on preventing and treating a higher-than-normal Blood sugar (remember your Bs).

For some reason, the idea of sugar "feeding" prostate and other cancers has been around a long time. However, it's a misunderstood situation because consuming sugar is not the actual issue. The reality is a high blood sugar or insulin level (pre-diabetes or diabetes) could increase the risk of being diagnosed with cancer, increase the side effects of some cancer treatments, and could (theoretically) increase the risk of cancer progression, or cancer retuning after treatment. Consuming some sugar in food should not be the focus because eating too many calories from any source (e.g., alcohol, sugar, fat, protein) and being more physically inactive may cause unhealthy weight/

waist gain that could lead to insulin resistance (higher insulin levels) and higher blood sugar, which theoretically could encourage cancer growth. If cancer progression was just about not consuming some sugar from beverages or food, then cancer would have been solved long ago. Proof can also be seen in both newer and older PET/CT scans, which exploit the ability of cancer cells to absorb the building blocks of fats, proteins, sugar, and countless other products. During the scan, the cancer consumes an artificially made compound that looks exactly like a building block of fat, protein, or sugar, and this allows the scan to precisely locate cancer and light this area up on the screen. Additionally, the human body (liver) needs to always produce a certain quantity of blood glucose (building block of sugar) for the brain and the rest of the body to survive. So, to fight cancer should you not eat anything? Of course not. Instead, do not let an excess of food or beverages, or any aspect of your lifestyle cause unhealthy increases in any of your B numbers, and that includes this fourth B (glucose).

This is precisely why the Bs are so powerful—because they help you and your healthcare team evaluate how you're doing with your diet and other aspects of your lifestyle. There should be an "emphasis" on just eating and being healthier to keep your stress levels low, rather than an "obsession" with eating and being healthier, which can increase your stress levels, and is not evidence-based. Again, let the Bs and your healthcare team guide you in the right direction.

PW Lifestyle Empowerment Moment

First Step: Lifestyle Changes Change Lives

DPP should have solidified a Nobel prize for lifestyle changes.

The clinical trial named the Diabetes Prevention Program (DPP) should have launched a lifestyle revolution, but instead it appeared to make a very good drug even more popular. The DPP trial was published in the *New England Journal of Medicine* way back in 2002. This clinical trial included 3,234 non-diabetic individuals who were at a high-risk for type 2 diabetes (prediabetes). The participants were randomly assigned either to a placebo, the drug metformin twice daily (850 mg for first month then 850 mg twice a day thereafter), or lifestyle changes with a goal of at least 7% weight loss (via a low-calorie, low-fat diet) with 150 minutes of physical activity per week. The average age of participants was 51 years old and on-average the participants were obese, although approximately 33% of the participants were of normal weight or overweight. A total of 68% were women, 45% of the members were minorities, and 20% were 60 years of age or older. Approximately 70% of the participants had a family history of diabetes and 16% of the women had a history of gestational diabetes. The average follow-up was only 2.8 years because the findings were so stunning within such a short period of time!

When the results were analyzed, compared to placebo, the group taking metformin reduced the risk of diabetes by 31%, but the lifestyle-intervention group reduced the risk by a whopping 58%! It turned out that lifestyle intervention was significantly more effective than metformin. Overall, the results did not significantly differ by gender, race, or ethnic group. The total daily caloric intake was reduced by 249 calories in the placebo group, 296 in the metformin group, and by 450 calories in the lifestyle group. The average weight loss was 0.1 kg (0.2

pounds), 2.1 kg (4.6 pounds), and 5.6 kg (over 12.3 pounds) in the placebo, metformin, and lifestyle groups, respectively. Interestingly, side effects with metformin were significantly greater than placebo in terms of gastrointestinal symptoms (i.e., diarrhea, flatulence, nausea, and vomiting). Not surprisingly, side effects for those in the lifestyle group were significantly lower than metformin.

After following some of participants in the DPP trial for 10 years, it appears that the results overall continue to stand the test of time with lifestyle changes still besting metformin, but both clearly reducing the risk of type 2 diabetes. Metformin, a primarily generic low-cost drug, has received a good deal of attention for the results demonstrated in the study. Imagine if a high-risk individual needing metformin also practiced some of the intensive lifestyle changes used by that group. Could the results be even more dramatic? I think so!

Still, consider how powerful the results of the DPP study are—lifestyle changes alone can reduce the risk of developing diabetes by almost 60%! In the participants ages 60 and older it reduced the risk of diabetes by over 70%! And research today from surgical weight loss or lifestyle changes are demonstrating that some individuals with type 2 diabetes can slow the progression, reverse, or eliminate their diabetes with proper diet and weight loss. Even individuals genetically predestined to end up getting type 2 diabetes might be able delay the onset by years, or even decades, in some cases! The bottom line is lifestyle changes can have a powerful impact in controlling diabetes. For even more information, please go to diabetes.org/are-you-at-risk/diabetes-risk-test to take a diabetes risk test from the American Diabetes Association and share these results with your healthcare team. Keep in mind that new research suggests higher hemoglobin A1c could also be predictive of a higher risk of cardiovascular disease in some individuals.

Second Step: Several low-cost medications in addition to lifestyle changes can change lives and possibly reduce certain side effects of some prostate cancer treatments.

The good news is there is a long list of potentially effective, low-cost medications used to control or reduce blood glucose today. Metformin, for example, which was mentioned earlier is not only one of the lowest cost glucose controlling medications, but it's also being studied in earlier stages of prostate cancer and with androgen deprivation therapy (ADT) to see if it could be used (in addition to conventional medicine) to treat prostate cancer, or at least reduce some of the side effects of ADT (e.g., weight gain, blood glucose increases). Other medications, such as semaglutide (mentioned in Appendix 1), which were originally used to control blood sugar in some patients with type 2 diabetes have also been approved to help with weight loss in a variety of individuals. Talk to your healthcare team about which options may be right for you.

PW Lifestyle Empowerment Moment

Medications to block the absorption of sugar (acarbose), or to push sugar into the urine (SGLT inhibitors), or to reduce the amount of sugar the body makes (metformin), and/ or reducing your exposure to bad sugars through newer medications (semaglutide), but also of course, dietary and other lifestyle changes increase your health investment portfolio by 100 times?!

Interestingly, in some parts of the world a group of older medications known as "alpha-glucosidase inhibitors" (acarbose, etc.) have been popular for some time for those with prediabetes and type 2 diabetes, and these pills are used at the beginning of each major meal of the day. These medications work by temporarily blocking the enzymes in the small intestine that help in the digestion of many complex carbohydrates into simple sugars (for example glucose, but it has minimal-to-no impact on the breakdown of lactose), so less sugar is absorbed from meals over time. These medications not only resulted in some weight loss, but also a lower risk of some cardiovascular events.

There is another class of newer medications (SGLT2 inhibitors) for diabetics that help push sugar out of the body and into the urine, which have also resulted in some weight loss, and a reduction in cardiovascular events. Part of the reason low-carbohydrate dieting (LCD) has also demonstrated some interesting preliminary results in improving the metabolic health of some prostate cancer patients (as has multiple other diet plans) is essentially utilizing the same concept, which is reducing the body's exposure to carbohydrates (sugars), but without blocking any of the intestinal enzymes or removing existing sugar from the body into the urine. Another similar concept in dieting involves consuming low glycemic index (GI) foods, which also reduces the body's exposure to unhealthy carbohydrates such as processed foods, fast-foods, sugar-containing beverages, etc. and getting more healthy plant-based carbohydrates (veggies, fruit, beans, lentils, etc. but also protein and fat). Studies using some of these diets in certain prostate cancer patients with and without some of these and other glucose controlling medications (metformin for example reduces the liver's production of glucose) have already demonstrated beneficial effects in improving various aspects of metabolic health, including weight loss, or reducing the side effects of treatment (ADT, etc.). The moral of the story is the history of effective or successful medications for those with pre-diabetes, or even type 2 diabetes have demonstrated that many were first heart healthy (our mantra), resulted in weight loss (1stB), and controlled or reduced the 4thB, which then could improve other Bs!

Even the newest heart healthiest weight loss drug on the market (semaglutide) causes someone to eat less, because it slows down how fast the stomach empties (so you just eat less of most things). So, is it really a surprise that reducing your exposure to excessive amounts of calories from simple sugars, including through diet and not just medications, has resulted in such profound heart, metabolic, and potentially other health benefits for prostate cancer patients by controlling or reducing the 4thB, which then results in multiple benefits for the other Bs?! (See the diet chapter please!)

What also gets missed in the history lesson are the benefits of exercise in controlling or reducing blood sugar. As the body becomes more fit aerobically, and through an increase in lean muscle mass via resistance activities then the chances of further improving your 4th B increases significantly because not only is less insulin needed, but more glucose is utilized by the muscles. Research suggests glucose uptake is up to 100 times greater when the body is exercising compared to being at rest! Now who doesn't want an investment with a 100-fold return? Lifestyle changes can change lives, but by also reducing the side effects of prostate cancer treatment via the 4thB!

Metabolic Syndrome (MetS) and metabolic health can now be introduced to you because you know the first B's!

There is accumulating research demonstrating the potential for metabolic syndrome (MetS) to be unhealthy for men (and women), because it may encourage the progression of prostate enlargement (BPH), prostate cancer, the side effects of cancer treatment, and cause erectile dysfunction (ED). However, MetS is currently much better recognized globally as a group of five risk factors or conditions (numbers) that can increase the risk of CVD (e.g., heart attack, stroke) and diabetes. Isn't it incredible how heart health and prostate health continue to be associated, especially in terms of similar increased or decreased risks?!

Metabolic syndrome requires the presence of at least three of the following five criteria listed in the next table. If you've read the first few chapters of this book, you'll recognize all of them. If you're at risk for MetS or have been diagnosed with MetS please review the first four chapters of this book with your healthcare team and realize that it can be controlled or reversed with lifestyle changes and medications (if needed). Again, lifestyle changes change lives, and they make medications work better at lower dosages, if you need a medication.

Metabolic Syndrome (MetS) Criteria: At least 3 of 5 are needed to be diagnosed with this condition:

Metabolic Syndrome Criteria	Specific Numbers Needed
Triglycerides ("fat in the blood")	Greater than 150 mg/dL (1.7 mmol/L)
HDL ("good cholesterol")	Less than 40 mg/dL (1.0 mmol/L) (For women—less than 50 mg/dL or 1.3 mmol/L)
Glucose ("fasting blood sugar")	Greater than 100 mg/dL (5.55 mmol/L)
Waist Circumference (WC)	Greater than 40 inches (102 cm) (For women—greater than 35 inches or 89 cm)
Blood Pressure (BP)	Greater or equal to 130/85

Note: *Some authoritative groups have slightly different requirements or numbers, but in general these are the commonly accepted criteria. MetS is associated with androgen deprivation treatment (ADT) for example, because a loss of testosterone can increase the risk of this syndrome, especially if lifestyle changes and possible medication assistance is not emphasized.*

This is another reason the 5 Bs are so critical to know, follow, and improve on with lifestyle changes and medications (if needed). The first chapter of this book reviewed waist circumference, the second chapter covered triglycerides and HDL, the third chapter covered blood pressure, and this chapter discussed glucose (and the hemoglobin A1c test), all of which contribute to metabolic syndrome. Whether you have "MetS" or are just more aware of the B's and how they impact your overall health, the best way to end this chapter is another critical reminder that hearth healthy = prostate healthy = head-to-toe healthier for men and women!

Appendix 5—The Fifth B = Brain Health

Brain Healthy = Head-to-Toe Healthier

Cancer is a "couple's condition" (you and your partner are in this together).

Before we discuss any aspect of a patient's mental health, we must first look at something that can easily get missed: the mental and physical impact on the caregiver or primary partner of the person diagnosed with cancer. Decades of research continues to suggest both individuals in any strong partnership, relationship, or marriage have the potential to be mentally and sometimes physically impacted to a similar degree. In other words, one person has been diagnosed, is being treated or has been treated for cancer, but the stress and other mental and physical health impacts are being shared equally or distributed between the partners. "Cancer is a couple's condition" (arguably my favorite teaching point), which means both partners need to make sure their physical and mental health is a priority during this time. That's why we made sure all the Bs in this book, as well as most of the other information (e.g., diet, exercise, sleep) is helpful if you have cancer, or are the person(s) taking care of someone with cancer. Again, cancer is a couple's condition. Take care of each other, prioritize each other, and just as important, please celebrate each other!

Please talk about the S.A.D. things with your healthcare team.

Mental health is an area that always needs more attention during cancer treatment. While we tend to focus on the physical aspects, it is very important to discuss issues such as stress, anxiety, and/or depression with your healthcare team. I refer to these mental issues as S.A.D., an acronym I have written about in the past (and an easy way to remember to discuss these three specific issues with your healthcare team). Without proper physical health it's challenging to maintain positive mental health, and without being in the best mental health it's tough to appreciate and strive for better physical health. There is also an association between mental health and heart health. Studies show that poor mental health can increase the risk of being heart unhealthy, but the good news is it works both ways: Improved mental health can enhance your heart health.

The brain is simply symbolic of mental health because communication with brain cells and various compounds or neurotransmitters (for example, serotonin) could impact mental fitness, but we recognize this is a simplistic way of looking at this issue. S.A.D. and any other aspects of brain health are impacted by a wide range of things (e.g., environment, genetics, lifestyle, medical conditions) that your healthcare team is far more qualified to address than any book.

Stress, anxiety, and depression (S.A.D.) are arguably the least-appreciated areas of medicine because there is still so much historical stigma attached to mental health issues. In the past (and still today), some patients, partners, family members, and even some healthcare providers are reluctant to talk about these issues. **We need to appreciate the importance of better mental health in promoting better physical (heart) health and better physical (heart) health in promoting better mental health.** The Brain B is a barometer that's just as important as all the other barometers, especially in individuals dealing with cancer.

Thankfully, there are many ways your healthcare team can evaluate your risk or progress when dealing with stress, anxiety, depression, or any other mental health issues. For example, there are many informative questionnaires used to diagnose depression, as well as comprehensive assessments on how stress or anxiety are impacting you. Additionally, there are many options today for treating mental issues, from lifestyle changes and therapy to other medical interventions.

During regular visits with your healthcare team, you want to be sure that it's not only a discussion about your physical health, but also your mental health. If you're not sure how to begin this dialogue, you can use the following list as a guide or conversation starters about issues directly or indirectly impacting various aspects of mental health:

- Level of sadness
- Level of happiness
- Future optimism or confidence
- Satisfaction out of daily life
- Level of control you have over your life
- How you perceive yourself physically and mentally
- Current perception of your overall physical and mental health
- How you think others perceive you physically and mentally
- Level of interest in life
- Level of worry or concern in your life
- Level of stress and/or anxiety
- Mood in general and in specific situations
- General and specific pain
- Skin and other health status
- Sleep habits
- Eating habits
- Energy level
- Other health concerns (weight loss/gain, gain, self-medications, etc.)
- Sexual health concerns
- Family situation or benefits and stressors
- Work satisfaction or benefits and stressors
- Primary or current support network

There are so many ways to communicate your mental and physical health to your medical team. In addition to the list above, you may also consider showing your healthcare team your latest journal entries. Either way, having these important discussions can make a profound difference in your overall health, both now and in the future. PLEASE be strong and take advantage of this barometer of health for a better and beautiful life. **It's also empowering to consider bringing your partner to your medical visits, if possible, especially when dealing with or evaluating your mental health.** He or she may be able to convey a different perspective to your healthcare team in terms of how your specific or overall mental health has been doing over time (improving or not improving). They may also be able to help you review and remember some of the things discussed by your healthcare team during your visit.

Further increasing S.A.D. awareness and discussions before, during and after any cancer treatment is one of the most important goals of this chapter and this entire book series!

Wellness is a wonderful word, and promoting wellness are two words reflecting hope and optimism, but mental health wellness and awareness must be as important as any other B! If this is true than we (our writing, editing, and publishing team) need to practice what we preach and discuss it more right here and now! This especially important when you've been diagnosed with cancer since the diagnosis itself increases the risk of mental health challenges. Going through treatment, or even non-treatment, recovery, or dealing with short or long-term side effects are not just physically challenging, but also mentally difficult. Research and patient advocacy have shed light on topics that had received minimal attention in the past.

For example, in prostate cancer anxiety and depression impact a large percentage of men within the first decade after diagnosis, and most men with advancing disease deal with stress or emotional distress at some point in the process. Recent interesting research from commercial and Medicare Advantage health plans found that among men diagnosed with anxiety or depression after initiating ADT, almost half do not receive mental health treatment. In addition, the use of counseling forms of therapy occurred in less than 1% of the men receiving treatment!

Medications were utilized in some cases, but most mental health prescriptions "originated" from primary care providers (not specialists), and though many were intended for short-term use of anxiety (e.g., benzodiazepine drugs), many patients used these medications chronically (or long-term). Some of these short-term medications have the potential for dependency, and can increase the risk of cognitive issues, as well as falls and bone breaks. In other words, men with some of these mental health issues (whether they have cancer or not) need more specialized forms of evaluation and treatment. Treatment should be better individualized, and more appropriate prescription medications (intended for longer-term use) should be prescribed, when needed.

Past studies from Veterans and Medicare databases have also found an increased risk of these types of mental health challenges in prostate cancer patients. ADT utilization is an important health marker for research in these situations, because first it suggests someone is currently dealing with prostate cancer, and they are also at a potentially higher risk for locally advanced, or advanced cancer. Additionally, they are typically dealing with the common and not so common short and long-term side effects of ADT, along with the added effects of other medications used with ADT today. Any, some, or all of these treatment scenarios can be mentally challenging. The multitude of available options (i.e., active surveillance, surgery, radiation, focal treatment, newer anti-androgens, chemotherapy, immune enhancement, PARP inhibitors, radio-ligand, radiopharmaceuticals, imaging, biomarkers, etc.) today should be personally encouraging and a reason for optimism, but these options are also daunting. So, this is not just about ADT, but the diagnosis, non-treatment, and all other treatments for prostate cancer.

Primary care management of a patients on ADT, or even going through some of the issues associated with other cancer treatments, may be a starting point but it cannot be where mental health advocacy completely stops. If this is an indication of what is occurring in the world outside of cancer treatment than there is much work to be done—which is more than enough reason to make mental (brain) health the 5th and one of the most important Bs in prostate cancer! We need to do better!

You and your partner can play your part by making sure you let your healthcare team know that mental health is as much your priority as your physical health. Seeing a specialist for cancer treatment is of course the expectation, or the rule and not the exception, but seeing a mental health specialist appears to still be the exception and not the rule. Let your healthcare team know if they, you, your partner, or primary care provider thinks you need more help in this area, because just like your physical treatment, you need to express that you would be open to seeing a specialist for your mental health treatment (if needed). I believe that today's healthcare teams (oncologists, urologists, nurses, social workers, primary care, physician assistants, etc.), in general, embrace the idea of referring or helping you get the help you need. However, with such intense passion for physical treatment success today and the number of options available, I also believe it can be easier than ever to miss the other side of treatment success!

PW Lifestyle Empowerment Moment

Lifestyle changes are one of the many important pieces in solving your puzzle.

What probably gets missed more than any other barometer of health is the sheer amount of research that now suggests how lifestyle changes, including diet and exercise, can prevent and/or improve some forms of depression, stress, and anxiety along with conventional treatment. In fact, there is now good research to suggest that the chances of experiencing remission from depression, for example, are greater in individuals that combine medical treatment with regular exercise and other positive lifestyle changes. The added advantage of lifestyle changes is that it allows you to work with your healthcare team to be on the most appropriate and safest dose of medication for effectiveness.

Lifestyle changes not only continue to reduce some of the potential side effects of these medications, but again can improve their effectiveness. For example, recent evidence from the ERASE randomized trial of prostate cancer patients found significant improvements in self-esteem, and significant reductions in the following: stress, prostate cancer-specific anxiety, fear of progression, and fatigue in the exercise group (just 3 times/week) vs. the control group, and all these benefits occurred within 12-weeks! Lifestyle changes change lives!

At the beginning of this book, we discussed the importance of collecting puzzle pieces to arrive at the right destination for you—solving your puzzle with your healthcare team to increase the chances of living longer and better. This requires looking at many pathways or options, which will ultimately work together to give you the results you need. Mental health, like any other medical condition, is more likely to benefit when approached in the same way. Addressing lifestyle changes, environmental situation, genetics, working closer with your healthcare team, asking for help, therapy, medication needs or changes...all these pathways are important.

5BBs (Bonus Barometers for better Head-to-Toe Health.)

The next few pages discuss "Bonus Bs" that are also critically important for overall mental and physical health. Some are as important as the Bs we have already covered and some less so, depending on the individual. Regardless, the 5BBs portion of this book can help increase the chances that you will experience head-to-toe health working with your healthcare team. Please enjoy the list because it was not easy coming up with all these B words, but it sure was fun and motivational when we completed this list!

Appendix 5B—The Bonus Barometers (BB'S)

Bonus B Health = Head-to-Toe Healthier

Beyond the handful of B's we've already discussed, there are many other "barometers" that provide better insight into your overall health. Feel free to review these with your healthcare team and add any additional barometers they suggest or that you find make a difference in your life and how you feel. (They don't have to start with B, but of course we like it when they do—but we don't want to Be-labor this point.)

Bonus Barometer (Behaviors) Checklist	What this Barometer Means
Batteries (CO, Fire Detector, etc.)	How many more injuries or deaths from carbon monoxide (CO) and from fires in the home could be prevented yearly with updated working alarm detectors? Please check your batteries in any of these CO or fire detectors because basically all of them need to be replaced every 6 months-to-1 year (& tested even more often). Also, always clean dust and debris off your detectors. Brief periodic alarm chirps are annoying, but it's your alarm begging for its batteries to be replaced!
Beats (RHR, EKG, CAC, CTA, CUS, etc.)	Your resting heart rate (RHR) is another excellent indicator of your heart health and fitness because greater fitness results in a lower RHR (heart muscle is stronger), or one that does not increase much over time. It's why runners for example, have such low RHRs. Make sure your medical team knows your average RHR. Also, applications (Apps) attached to your cell phone can now take an EKG (ECG) to not only accurately measure RHR, but also detect abnormal heart rhythms such as "atrial fibrillation."

Beats (RHR, EKG, CAC, CTA, CUS, etc.) cont.	Get one if your healthcare team thinks it's a good idea for you. (One example is "KardiaMobile," but there are many others.) CT coronary artery calcium score—"CAC" (and in some cases the CT coronary angiogram—"CTA") for select intermediate or undetermined cardiovascular risk patients is also becoming more used by medical teams in cases where a clearer picture of heart health or heart disease risk is needed. Even a carotid ultrasound (CUS), or other tests, could be useful in some select individuals if your medical team thinks you are a candidate.
Bedtime (SEE SLEEP TIPS AT THE END OF THIS SECTION)	Sleep: How much (quantity) shuteye are you getting, and is it good quality? Do you snore? Are you waking up tired? Are you falling asleep with your TV/tech on? Poor sleep impacts a variety of health conditions, not least of which are increased risk of weight gain and increased blood pressure and blood sugar. (Too much sleep isn't good for you either.) Recent amazing evidence suggests one of the many reasons we need sleep is it allows the brain to clear debris or metabolic junk via what is known as the "glymphatic system," which could otherwise be harmful to the brain in long-term sleep deprived individuals.
Beliefs	Religion/Spirituality: You and your healthcare team should embrace and respect your religious or spiritual beliefs. Having a strong spiritual outlet does help some patients mentally and physically.

Beneficence (Benevolent & Beautiful)	Charity, volunteering, concern, and kindness towards others seems selfless, but research has demonstrated it's also wonderfully selfish, so to speak by often improving the mental and physical well-being of the person giving their time to others. Support groups, helplines, etc. There are so many ways people impacted by cancer (both patients and caregivers) give their time and experience to others that it's one of the most incredible acts of humanity I have had the privilege of witnessing during my entire career. Beneficence is benevolent and beautiful!
"Better Half" (or just other half)	Just another reminder that cancer is a couple's condition, so make sure you and your better half are looking out for each other's mental and physical health during this time. In a true partnership health is a two-way street!
Bills (Bank)	Financial stress/toxicity/volatility/instability continues to demonstrate from recent studies that it can have a profound impact on your mental and/or physical health. If there are issues with this B (Barometer) please seek assistance by talking to your healthcare team, including a social worker. They may be able to reduce direct and indirect medical costs, and other financial (or non-financial) burdens you could be experiencing right now.
Bite	Dental health: Gum inflammation and infection may impact certain diseases and vice versa: Certain conditions and/or medications (for osteoporosis treatment) can make you more susceptible to dental issues and infections. Talk to your healthcare team about how to prevent these problems. Dental healthy = Heart healthy!

Bites	Diet: The quality and quantity (QQ) of your diet (aka dietary pattern) is as important as any other aspect of your health.
Blood flow (Brain & Below)	Periodic cognitive testing in some individuals is more common today, and keep in mind exercise is one of the best ways to improve blood flow to the brain and below! Sexual health (erectile function) and sexual drive (libido) are important barometers of your overall health. In men, erectile dysfunction (ED), for example could also be an early indication of less optimal heart health.
Bloodline, BRCA-1 or BRCA-2 (genetics/family history), **B12** or other **Blood work**	Family health tree (aka family disease tree): Charting first-degree relatives' (parents, siblings, and children) medical conditions and/or their specific cause of death can shed light on your genetic and other risk factors. For example, BRCA-1 and BRCA-2 mutations not only increase the potential risk of breast and ovarian cancer in women, but also prostate and potentially other cancers, and more aggressive disease in some men, so some men need a BRCA-1 and BRCA-2 test now (talk to your medical team)! In addition, weight gain or loss, a primarily plant-based diet, and some common medications (acid reflux pills, metformin, etc.), surgical procedures, etc. can lower vitamin B12 levels, so ask if you need this or another blood test, including a complete blood count, metabolic profile, or even in some cases vitamin D levels. Other blood tests should also be discussed with your healthcare team. BRCA-1 and BRCA-2 for example can also be tested by a cheek swab or blood.

Body & Brain Building (Brawny & Blissfully Bold)	Exercise: Aerobic, flexibility and resistance (strength) forms of physical activity are as important as any other aspect of your health. Research continues to demonstrate that mind-body type exercise (Meditation, Tai Chi, Qigong, Pilates, Yoga, etc.) provide mental and physical health benefits in cancer patients!
Boosters (SEE VACCINES LATER IN THIS CHAPTER)	Vaccines: Compliance with adult vaccines, from COVID-19 and flu to pneumonia, shingles, tetanus, and others identified by your healthcare team, are critical for a healthier heart and overall health. In fact, recent research suggests that some adult vaccines could reduce the risk of CVD events (heart attack, stroke, etc.), potentially reduce or better control inflammation, and could provide a variety of other unappreciated health benefits.
Booze	Alcohol intake: Excessive consumption of alcohol can increase weight, inflammation, atrial fibrillation (AF), and the risk of infections. It can also increase the risk of aggressive cancer, and the risk of cancer returning after treatment. Even minimal-to-moderate consumption in some individuals is associated with worsening mental and physical health.

Bowel, Bone, Breast (primarily in women but also in some select men with a strong history-BRCA1 or BRCA2), and **Basic Body Barometers** (Screenings)	Screenings for other cancers and conditions (osteoporosis, etc.): Colonoscopies or other colon cancer screenings (starting at age 45 years now), one time (at the very least) hepatitis C screening, and periodic bone density DEXA screenings, especially if you are starting or on androgen deprivation therapy (ADT) for prostate cancer, can help you stay healthier from head-to-toe. For example, when it comes to bone health, the FRAX questionnaire/score (it's just 12 questions and is typically used after you get a DEXA bone density scan) can give you an idea of your 10-year risk of experiencing a bone fracture (look it up at sheffield.ac.uk/FRAX). Which other conditions you qualify for right now, or in the future, should be discussed with your healthcare team (e.g., hearing, vision, skin cancer) because these are personal decisions.
Boys (and of course girls and anyone else in your inner or outer circle)	One of the most underappreciated aspects of any cancer diagnosis is what you can tell your children, other family members and friends, and anyone else in your circle, to potentially avoid dealing with what you had to deal with. This is a tough one, but many prostate, breast, and ovarian cancers do not have an obvious cause. However, what we do know (apart from genetic testing when needed such as BRCA-1, BRCA-2, Lynch Syndrome and others) is trying to do "whatever you can to reduce your cardiovascular risk to as close to zero as possible" is arguably the best advice you can give anyone, including your boys and girls, to help them live their longest and best life (yes, it all goes back to the Bs!). What is your son's, daughter's, partner's or best friend's BMI, blood cholesterol, blood pressure, blood sugar, brain health, and other Bs? Use this book not just for yourself, but please pay this information forward. This is what the boys/men in your family and anyone else should know.

Broad-Brimmed (Bucket) & **Balm** to **Block** (But not Baseball?!)	How many cases of skin cancers (and premature wrinkling/aging) could be prevented by regularly using broad-brimmed hats (or even bucket or legionnaire-style ones) to block out ultraviolet light (UVA & UVB)? Baseball caps, although better than nothing, allow too much sun exposure especially of the ears (cancer happens there too), but also the cheeks, nose and neck. Also, select your sunscreen carefully because I believe the "physical" (aka "mineral," zinc oxide, titanium dioxide) sunscreens are outstanding since they are usually cost-effective, work the moment you apply them, are safe for environment (i.e., coral reefs—check labels), can be healthy for the skin in general, and you do not absorb much or any of it into your bloodstream (unlike many of the more expensive "chemical" sunscreens, which the FDA determined could be more absorbed into the body than originally believed). Don't forget to do your homework on sunglasses, sun-protective clothing, and lip balm (the forgotten area of the face), and always seeking shade for sun relief. In Australia there is a wonderful campaign called the Slip, Slop, Slap, Seek, and Slide (google it please) to remind all of us to do these important things.
Buddies	Support network: Whether it's working closely with your partner (cancer is a couple's condition as mentioned earlier) or belonging to a group that meets in person regularly or sharing your experience with people on the internet, increasing your social network can be both therapeutic and educational. (Be careful though: Constantly hearing about other people's losses via online social networks can increase your stress level in some cases, which is what some research refers to as the "cost of caring." Cost of caring also refers to "compassion fatigue" where one partner or cancer patient is constantly trying to make things better for another person at the cost of their own health.)

Buddies that Bark (Bowwow...)	Research continues to suggest the physical and mental health benefits of owning a pet (from a bowwow to a meow and others), whether it's increased physical activity, companionship or even a reduction in cognitive decline or preserving mental health. In fact, even the Center for Disease Control (CDC) lists the following health benefits of pets: • Lower BP • Lower Blood cholesterol • Reduced feelings of loneliness • Increased opportunities for exercise and outdoor activities • Increased opportunities for socialization Wow! Sorry, I meant "Woof!"
Butts	Tobacco use: Current or past tobacco use, from cigarettes, smokeless tobacco, and even second-hand smoke can compromise your mental and physical health, worsen any medical treatments you're undergoing, and increase inflammation. Just please don't do it.
Buzz	Energy/fatigue level: Constant fatigue can be a sign of underlying hormonal or endocrine issues that should be evaluated by your healthcare team. Cancer-related fatigue (CRF) is a real issue today in some people. A healthy diet and regular exercise can boost energy without relying on artificial means. Also talk to your healthcare team (as always)!

	Suggestions from my partner/caregiver, medical team, and me (meaning "you"):
Other Bonus B's ("find health where you did not know it existed"—one of my favorite teaching mantras!)	One of my teaching points is to **"find health where you did not know it existed."** Everyone is similar, but also unique in what could help them become healthier. For example, less car commuting to work and more biking or walking, learning to cook, taking a dance class, doing more household chores, vacationing more, taking a yoga class, or joining a pickle ball team, bowling team, or bridge club...there is something in all of us initially not recognized by those in your outer circle that can help to make you mentally and/or physically healthier. What is that thing for you? There are many other underappreciated Bs just waiting to be discovered by you and others around you and that is part of what makes life so very beautiful!

Dr. M's Better Quality and Quantity (QQ) Sleep Tips (aka Bedtime Barometer)

Another topic that deserves more attention is sleep. It's something that most of us take for granted, but the quantity and quality (QQ) of sleep can have a tremendous impact on our health. For instance, humans tend to consume more processed foods and just more calories when they cannot sleep because "the longer you stay awake the greater the chance you will eat that piece of cake" (that rhymes), candy, chips, cookies, or crackers. Is this part of the reason getting less sleep increases the risk of some health problems including insulin resistance? Possibly, as found in the most recent research on sleep. Studies show that "weekend catch up sleep," from not getting enough shuteye during the work week, does not appear to be enough to solve insulin resistance issues from a lack of sleep.

Better quality and quantity (QQ) of sleep also carries a variety of health benefits, some of which are just beginning to be appreciated. For example, sleep allows for the more efficient cleansing of the waste or "trash" within the brain that is produced daily in large amounts. Because the brain requires such an incredible amount of energy to function during the day, it produces metabolic by-products. The "glymphatic system" naturally removes these potentially harmful by-products during the sleep cycle. Sleep research continues to suggest one of the best ways to keep the brain healthy and youthful is to be heart healthy and this includes improving the QQ of your sleep.

So, we decided to include some of my favorite research tips on how to improve your sleep QQ. It's a little corny, but it should be fun to read all the rhymes. Please keep in mind that these tips are useful regardless of where you are in your better sleep journey. In the same way that diet and exercise can help you whether you're using medications or receiving treatments or not, better sleep can do the same. Recent research continues to suggest many cancer patients have difficulty sleeping, and even some common treatments can disrupt sleep or increase the risk of insomnia, and when this occurs it can increase daily fatigue and even cognition. So, we decided it was time to add more updated sleep advice thanks to your letters or recommendations from past editions of these books. Thank you. Again, it may be a silly table, but the recommendations are evidenced-based and very serious.

Dr. M's silly, but serious sleep rhymes to improve your QQ without first relying on pills!	Commentary and Recommendations
"Block out all the outside light, primarily at night, so you can sleep tight." "In fact, even while you are getting some ZZZs new research suggests exposure to any light could be bad for your 5Bs!"	Block light in your room as much as possible because darkness promotes melatonin secretion. This includes darker and thicker curtains if possible. New research even suggests light exposure while sleeping can negatively impact heart and metabolic health.

"Turn off all the screens so that the wonders of natural melatonin can be seen (actually felt)."

Bright light and blue light from the TV, computers, cell phones and other screens can reduce melatonin production. Turn off screens and dim bedroom light 30 minutes before bedtime.

"Caffeine earlier in the day makes it easier to hit the hay, and before bed getting less alcohol and heavy food lets your body get into the best type of sleeping mood."

"Booze will not allow you to get a more salubrious snooze."

"And nicotine will keep you awake for goodness' sake (and it's heart unhealthy)!"

Caffeine can stay in some people's systems for many hours. Try and use it early in the day, so it does not disrupt your sleep. High food intake before bed can make you initially drowsy, but acid reflux from an excessive amount of food can keep you up. Alcohol helps you feel superficially sleepy, but it robs you of deep sleep. Also, no nicotine please!

"Increase your intake of plants to enhance your bedtime romance."

Is it really a surprise that new research suggests a healthier diet is associated with less sexual dysfunction and/or better sleep?! Where is that commercial?!

"Before taking any sleeping pill try your best to chill."

The National Sleep Foundation recommends keeping bedrooms at a cool 65 degrees Fahrenheit (18.3 degrees Celsius) for optimal sleep (slightly above or below that temperature is also commonly recommended). Too hot and you can lose dream sleep (REM) and wake up during the night (too cold is not healthy either). A mattress cooling device may also help.

"Exercising almost every day helps keeps stress and the urologist away, or at least at bay."	Meditation, aerobic/resistance/ flexibility exercises have demonstrated the ability to place you in deeper, more refreshing sleep cycles at night, along with potentially being more efficient at emptying your bladder during the day, thus reducing the need to urinate more at night (nocturia).
"Healthier weight can help you wake up feeling great!" **"In fact, even less weight on your lap gives you the chance to drop that CPAP."**	Weight gain increases the risk of sleep apnea and other breathing problems, acid reflux, and many other conditions that can completely disrupt your QQ! However, the amazing news is a little bit of weight/waist loss can reverse these sleep issues!
"Noise machines are best when internal or external sounds cannot be put to rest."	White noise and similar machines help those with tinnitus (ringing in the ears) sleep better, or those bothered by external sounds. White noise may also help individuals who have a hard time quieting their mind.
"33% of your total life, so PAY more attention to buying the best personal equipment to reduce your sleeping strife!" (Note: "Equipment" means mattress, sheets, blankets/ covers, pajamas, etc.)	Many people are willing to buy an expensive car, house, dog, vacation, exercise equipment, etc., but hesitate to invest in quality sleep aids, such as mattresses. Yet, what else besides sleep occupies so much of your life? Research mattresses, pillows, cooling blankets, room darkening shades and other sleep aids, and spend more if needed. Consumer Reports or another non-biased group ranking of the best quality products for the price should be a priority.

"Adhesive Nasal strip (for example Breathe Right) are another simple investment tip!"	Make sure you get the right size for your nose. These simple aids have helped a lot of folks breathe easier and sleep better.
"Review your diet, OTC, and prescription pills because some of these things could be causing your mind to never sit still!"	OTC pills and prescription medications can, at times, be the cause of sleep issues. For example, in men's health, testosterone replacement can worsen sleep apnea in some patients. Steroids, nicotine replacement, decongestants, over exposure to thyroid hormone replacement, pills with caffeine or "natural" sources of caffeine (guarana, yerba mate, etc.), kola nut, chocolate with a higher percentage of cocoa, etc. can disrupt sleep.
"Sleep Study or Sleep tracker Apps will improve your ability to take better naps!"	There are now at-home sleep monitoring devices your doctor can prescribe if there are concerns you have sleep apnea. There are also new sleep apps, so spending the night in a study lab is no longer necessary for many people.
"Cognitive Behavioral Therapy (CBT) instead of a sleeping pill could do more than anything to allow your mind to be still, so if in any doubt then please let a sleep specialist check you out!" **"If you think some of the sleeping tips in this section were keen, then again talking to a sleep professional will further help your sleep hygiene!"**	CBT is an effective method to increase your sleep QQ without pills and there are also on-line options available! Sleep medicine is essentially a medical specialty today, which means your healthcare team has a variety of options, including referring or recommending some experts in this category (sleep savants). Awareness is no longer an issue in any medical specialty and seeking out the best sleep hygiene tips is the key to better QQ. We all agree good sleep = good mental and physical health!

Note: *Many other things can impact sleep where pills are not necessarily the solution, including stress, anxiety, depression, rumination, catastrophizing, and more (some forms of hormonal treatment for prostate cancer for example could disrupt sleep, which could then impact cognition)...which is why your healthcare team and sleep health professionals have become a powerful option today that more people need to utilize! Please ask for help because when was the last time you heard an adult say, "I sleep like a baby every night?" Most of us share many things, including issues with the QQ of our sleep.*

The Importance of Boosters/Vaccines—7 things to think about when discussing them with your healthcare team (aka Boosters Barometer)

One of the bonus B's that deserves a little more attention is "boosters." In fact, only 25-50% of adults are caught-up on their adult preventive vaccines. Research suggests prostate cancer and other types of patients have similar preventive vaccine compliance rates to the general population, which is surprising because I believe with greater awareness of the issue the adherence percentages would dramatically and immediately increase. Cancer patients are at higher risk of mild infections turning into more serious problems, which is what was observed with COVID-19. This is the primary issue and why greater attention should be given to this subject before, during, or after any prostate cancer treatment (surgery, radiation, ADT, anti-androgens, chemotherapy, etc.), so here we go! Let's consider seven critical reasons to talk to your healthcare team about getting your vaccines updated:

1. **Heart-healthy and all-healthy.
   Under-appreciated side benefits!**

   New research suggests vaccines reduce the risk of getting or dying from multiple diseases that aren't related to the vaccine itself. For example, there is new consistent research to suggest vaccines could reduce the risk of cardiovascular disease (CVD) by controlling short- and long-term inflammation that occurs when you get an infection. When a person gets a serious infection, such as the flu, pneumonia, or shingles, there is a large inflammatory response that can be detected even six months to a year after the infection subsides. This large inflammatory response can share some of the same pathways with heart disease and stroke and can make an existing problem even worse. Therefore, one of the greatest side benefits of vaccines is that they are indeed heart healthy! Even more, there is new research suggesting some adult vaccines could enhance the effects of certain cancer treatments, which is being tested in clinical trials right now, and research has already demonstrated some vaccines, such as hepatitis B, are associated with lower rates of liver cancer. HPV vaccines are not only associated with a lower rate of some types of cervical cancer, but also potentially head and neck, penile, anal, and several other cancers. This is part of the reason why some individuals may quality for this vaccine even in their early 40s today (it was previously only available for younger individuals).

Still, it's worth repeating, there is now plenty of research suggesting many adult vaccines have been associated with lower rates of cardiovascular events! In fact, a recent randomized trial of the flu vaccine against a placebo conducted in those who experienced a recent cardiovascular event (heart attack), primarily conducted in Europe (known as "IAMI" trial), demonstrated a reduced risk of another cardiac event and dying younger from all causes in those patients that received a flu vaccine.

While it's common to hear about the potential side effects of a medication, supplement, or vaccine, learning about the side benefits is rare. Few people ever hear about the potential side benefits to some treatments, including adult vaccines. In fact, those benefits are just beginning to be appreciated. In addition, preliminary research continues to demonstrate that someone who is not caught up on all their adult vaccines appear to have an increased probability of being diagnosed with other more severe infections. In other words, vaccines put your immune system on high alert, not just for one type of infection, but potentially many other types of infections.

Before we move on to the other six reasons there are many vaccines desperate for more awareness, discussion, or utilization in the prostate and overall cancer community. Below is a partial list of the ones often missed by many adults and some of their potential "side benefits" that receive little-to-no attention.

Adult Vaccines in need of more awareness (Adult compliance on average is generally between 25-50%. We can do better right now!)	Potential Side Benefit (Not definitive, but suggestive because of the apparent increased risk of these other conditions when not vaccinated)
COVID-19 (SARS-CoV-2)	Reduces the risk of cardiovascular disease (CVD) events (heart attack, stroke, etc.).
Flu (influenza)	Reduces the risk of CVD events because of the flu and the large inflammatory response when dealing with a severe infection.
Hepatitis A and/or B	Reduces the risk of liver injury/ damage and liver cancer itself in some cases with Hep B vaccine.
HPV (Human papillomavirus)	Reduction in the risk of numerous cancers in men and women (anal, head, neck/mouth, and throat, penile, rectal, vaginal, and vulvar). Some adults ages 27 though 45 may now qualify for this vaccine.

Pneumonia vaccines	Reduces the risk of CVD events.
Shingles (Herpes zoster non-live vaccine-recombinant-also known as "Shingrix")	Reduces the risk of CVD events, temporary or permanent vision loss (HZO or herpes ophthalmicus), debilitating nerve pain (post-herpetic neuralgia), rare PSA flare, etc. Some prostate cancer treatments have been associated with an increased risk of shingles perhaps due to stress or immune changes (another of the many reasons to be vaccinated). (Also, see note 3 below for recent finding regarding shingles and COVID-19.)
Tdap and/or Td booster	Tetanus can increase the risk of a cardiovascular event. The vaccine is being studied in human clinical trials against other cancers to potentially enhance the treatment effects of some conventional immune therapies.

Notes:

1. An antibody test from your healthcare team can help determine if you were exposed to an infectious agent in the past, such as chickenpox, since some people do not remember whether they had it as an adolescent or they could have been exposed or even infected with minimal-to-no symptoms (subclinical case).

2. Hepatitis A and/or B have multiple other situations where you can qualify. In addition, there is also the potential qualification for these vaccine(s) even though you are "not at risk but want protection from hepatitis A and/or B."

3. People 50 and older who have had a mild case of COVID-19 are 15% more likely to develop shingles (herpes zoster) within six month(s) than are those who have not been

infected by the coronavirus, according to research. However, the risk "was found to be even greater for older people who were hospitalized because of a more severe COVID case, making them 21% more likely to develop shingles than those who did not have COVID." These findings were published in Open Forum Infectious Diseases.

PW Lifestyle Empowerment Moment

Again, vaccines should be viewed as heart healthy because many of them appear to reduce the risk of CVD events (as outlined above), which can be caused by an infectious disease. COVID-19 has been the most obvious recent example of how an infectious or respiratory disease could also be viewed as a cardiovascular disease since it appears to increase the risk of inflammation of the heart, blood vessels, heart attack, stroke, blood clots, and more, especially in people more vulnerable or at risk, such as cancer patients. It's interesting how some COVID-19 vaccines received so much attention because they could rarely cause temporary heart inflammation in some individuals, but what failed to receive more attention was the severe and potentially deadly cardiovascular or heart inflammation consequences that could be caused by COVID-19 itself when someone was not protected by the vaccine.

It was also mentioned earlier in the book of how there is a prostate cancer treatment paradox, whereby some effective new and old medications used to treat this disease also have an ability to increase the risk of CVD. It's for this reason healthy behaviors and numbers are so critical, which includes getting caught up on the adult vaccines your healthcare team approves right now. It's also important to mention that the paradox of prostate cancer treatment also exists for some other cancers and infectious diseases. For example, getting malaria can raise the risk of numerous cardiovascular problems and many effective anti-malarial treatments also increase the risk of cardiovascular side effects. Malaria can cause inflammation of the heart, arrhythmias, heart failure, anemia, and other issues, and anti-malaria treatments have their own cardiovascular risks. In other words, we have known for some time that common infectious diseases throughout the world are potentially heart unhealthy and vaccinations for these diseases have been advertised as preventing these infections. But it seems more of the amazing potential side benefits or heart healthy advantages of these vaccines get lost in the discussion of why they are so beneficial, and/or perhaps these ancillary benefits are not known?

Keep in mind, COVID-19, influenza, or pneumonia are all in the top 10 causes of death in the U.S., and all three conditions are again known to raise the risk of cardiovascular problems. When you consider this, is it a surprise that all these vaccines could be heart healthy by preventing someone from getting or dealing with these infections in the first place? Finally, it's also interesting that many of the vaccines in the table have research now to suggest the more heart healthy you are through your behaviors (lifestyle) and numbers then the more effective the vaccine appears to be against these diseases! How about that for another reason to take care of yourself and be as heart healthy as possible! Lifestyle changes change lives!

2. They can dramatically lessen severity (reduce excessive inflammation) even when they do not completely prevent something.

Vaccines are designed to protect you from a life-threatening disease, but even if you still get that disease, it can reduce the severity, which could keep you out of the hospital (or worse). As an example, the shingles vaccine dramatically reduces your risk of experiencing long-term or severe post-herpetic neuralgia (PHN), debilitating nerve pain or even vision loss if shingles gets into the eye. You continue to have memory immune cells from your vaccines that help when battling a future illness. Just because you were unlucky enough to get the condition you were vaccinated against doesn't mean you won't directly benefit from it now or in the future. Reducing severity or even death from an illness was one of the least appreciated aspects of adult vaccines until COVID-19 vaccines became available. Of course, we now know vaccines to prevent severe COVID have a proven impressive track record. However, long before the COVID-19 pandemic, most adult vaccines were preventing countless individuals from being hospitalized or dying from the flu, pneumonia, and numerous other diseases.

3. The price is right!

Most vaccines are generally inexpensive for the patient, as most insurance companies will cover them under your plan. The cost is certainly reasonable in terms of what the vaccine can provide for you long-term (a better and longer life). Many periodic free health fairs, or awareness days even offer some adult vaccines. For example, I usually get my flu shot every year after giving a lecture at the free Men's Health Screening and Awareness Day at Ford Field, for example.

4. Let history be your lesson.

Vaccines are perhaps one of the greatest medical success stories in terms of saving lives and allowing people to enjoy a longer life. Arguably, nothing has saved more lives around the world than child and adult vaccinations.

5. Herd immunity.

Vaccines can provide "herd immunity," which can save the lives of people of all ages, especially the most immunologically vulnerable, such as the very young and old, and those with severe immune-suppressive diseases. Herd immunity occurs when enough individuals in a community get vaccinated so that there is little chance that a virus or bacteria can be transmitted to the most vulnerable individuals in the herd.

6. **Unlike the lottery, your odds of winning go up the sooner you play the game.**

   The sooner you get the vaccine, the better the potential result for you and those around you. All vaccines take time (approximately 2-4 weeks on average) to generate a response. Getting your vaccine early helps ensure you're fully ready to fight the illness. Additionally, there is a heightened immune surveillance, so early research on those vaccinated for other conditions appeared to provide protection against severe forms of COVID-19, for example.

7. **Please discuss the latest advantages of being vaccinated after being diagnosed and treated for cancer with your healthcare team.**

   Chemotherapy, androgen deprivation therapy (ADT), and even the stress of being diagnosed and treated for cancer can impact your immune system and has been associated with a higher risk of some stress-induced reactivating infections such as shingles, for example. Also, patients being treated for cancer simply have a higher risk of a mild infection becoming more severe. It's unimaginable how many more advantages will be found for cancer patients vaccinated against so many common infections, which is why just talking to your healthcare team about them is an added advantage because so many people do not take advantage of this wonderful opportunity.

<u>Congratulations you have now read all of the Bs from this Book and that's a Beautiful thing!</u> Now that you've completed the appendices on the 5 Bs & BBs (well, more than 5, but 5 sounds pithy), you have some measuring tools to help you move toward or maintain optimal health. If you find that you don't score as well as you'd like on those assessment tools just yet, don't be discouraged. **Please remember to always talk to and work with your medical team before making any changes to your healthcare plan, and thank** you for reading this book!